Osteoporosis Prevention

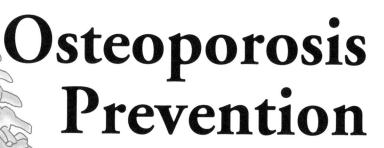

Osteoporosis Prevention

A *Proactive* Approach to Strong Bones and Good Health

RENÉE NEWMAN

 International Jewelry Publications
Los Angeles_____

International Jewelry Publications
P.O. Box 13384
Los Angeles, CA 90013-0384 USA

(Inquiries should be accompanied by a self-addressed,
stamped envelope.)

Printed in the United States of America

Library of Congress Cataloging-in-Publication Data

Newman, Renée.
   Osteoporosis prevention : a proactive approach to strong
bones and good health / Renée Newman.
       p. cm.
   Includes bibliographical references and index.
   ISBN-13: 978-0-929975-37-5
   ISBN-10: 0-929975-37-5
    1. Osteoporosis--Prevention. 2. Osteoporosis--Prevention
    –Popular works. I. Title.

   RC931.073N49 2006
   616.7'16–dc22

                                        2005047545

Cover design by Don Nelson
Cover artwork by Bonnie Nelson

To Mom,

A registered nurse who believed in the importance of preventing disease and communicating with patients—two themes of this book. During her final conversation with me in the hospital, she pointed to her RN and said "There's a really good nurse; she doesn't just hand you a pill; she tells you what it is, why you need it, and how it will help you."

Contents

Acknowledgments x

Preface xi

1 Why I decided to Write a Book on Osteoporosis 1
Why I Care More About My Bones Than the Average Person 2
Short Answers to Basic Questions about Osteoporosis 4

2 Density Versus Strength 9
Quiz: Chapters 1 & 2 11

3 Who is at Risk? 13
Osteoporosis Risk Factors You Cannot Change 13
Osteoporosis Risk Factors You Can Change 14
Diseases and Disorders that can Lead to Osteoporosis 16
Medications that can Cause Osteoporosis 17
Quiz: Chapter 3 19

4 Basic Bone Terminology 21
What is the Hip? 21
Spine Terms Found on Bone Density Reports 22
Basic Bone Terms 23
Quiz: Chapter 4 26

5 Making Exercise Safe and Fun 27
How We Know that Exercise Makes Bones Denser 27
What Types of Exercise are Good for Bones? 28
My Experiences With Four Types of Exercise 29
Bone-loading Activities for the Hip, Spine and Wrist 34
Choosing a Trainer 37
Making Exercise Fun 38
Incorporating Exercise Into Your Daily Activities 40
How to Help Seniors Maintain their Muscles & Bones 41
Quiz: Chapter 5 44

6   **Why I Volunteer in an Orthopedic Ward   47**

7   **Posture and Osteoporosis   49**
    Is Osteoporosis the Only Cause of Hunched Backs?   49
    How Easy is it to Have Good Posture?   50
    Tips for Having a Youthful Posture   51

8   **Calcium   53**
    How Do We Know That Calcium Helps Bone Growth?   53
    How Much Calcium Do People Need?   54
    How to Determine the Calcium Content of Food   55
    What Type of Calcium Supplement is Best?   58
    Substances that Reduce Calcium Absorption   60
    Substances that Cause Calcium Loss   61
    Guidelines for Consuming and Buying Calcium   62
    Consequences of Too Much Calcium   63
    Is Coral Calcium Better than other Calcium?   64
    Is Milk Bad for Bones?   65

9   **Other Bone Nutrients   67**
    Vitamin D   70
    Magnesium   71
    Vitamin K   73
    Boron   75
    Zinc   76
    Vitamin B_{12} 77
    Plant-derived Estrogens   79
    Nutrients that can be Both Good and Bad for Bones   81

10 **Fighting Osteoporosis and Losing Weight   83**
    Osteoporosis, Body Weight and Dieting   83
    Osteoporosis and Eating Disorders   84
    How I Lost Weight Fighting Osteoporosis   85
    How You can Lose Weight yet Get Adequate Nutrition   85
    A Wish List for Eating Out   86

11 **Osteoporosis Drugs: Pros & Cons   87**
    Taking Alendronate (Fosamax): A Personal Decision   87
    Why Take Bone Drugs Before You Have Osteoporosis?   88
    Why I've Never Taken Hormones   90
    "Natural" Hormones   91
    Some Criticisms and Advantages of Osteoporosis Drugs   92

12 Vibrating Platform Therapy 97

Promising Results for Lay People 98
Making Vibration Therapy Safe 99

13 Understanding Density Reports 101

What is a T-Score? 102
What is a Z-Score? 103
What's More Important: the T-Score or the Z-Score? 103
What's the Difference Between the T-score and BMD? 104

14 Bone Density Testing 105

Types of Bone Density Tests 105
Heel Tests Versus DXA Spine and Hip Tests 106
How Accurate are Bone Density Tests? 107
Who Should Be Tested? 110
Osteoporosis in Men 110
How Often Should People be Tested? 111
Contrasting Experiences With Bone Density Testing 113
Results of my Interviews About Bone Density Centers 113
Are Bone Density Tests Worthwhile? 114
Measuring Bone Turnover With Blood & Urine Tests 116

15 Side Benefits of Bone Density Tests 117

How Bone Density Tests Can Help You 117
Why Testing Centers Should Communicate with Patients 120
Why Technologists May Not Discuss Test Results 122
Jewelry Appraisals and Bone Appraisals 124
Paying for Bone Density Testing 126
Finding a Bone Density Center 126
What to Do if There's No DXA Center in Your Area 128
Should a Doctors's Order Be Required for DXA Tests? 128
Why You Should Study Your Density Reports Instead of Relying
    Solely on Your Doctors 129
How to Be a Savvy Patient 130

16 Pros & Cons of Giving Patients Their Medical Reports 133

Why Keeping Copies of Your Test Results Comes in Handy 133
Doctors' Concerns About Giving Patients Their Medical Reports 134
Doctors Who Show Patients Their Medical Reports 136

17 Hip and Spine DXA Tests: A Case Study 139
My Bone Density Exams 139
Four-year Study of the Changes in my Bone Densities 140
My Bone Density Data 144
Follow-up Visit with an Osteoporosis Specialist 152
Don't be Duped by Testimonials 153
Conclusions from This Four-year Study 155

18 How to Help Prevent Osteoporosis and Broken Bones 157
Diet 157
Physical Activity 158
Medications 161
Posture 162
Bone-Depleting Habits 162
Ten Major Causes of Falls & Broken Bones 163
More Tips for Avoiding Falls and Fractures 164
How to Help Others Maintain Strong Bones & Good Health 165

Osteoporosis Websites 167

Bibliography 169

Index 173

Acknowledgments

I would like to express my appreciation to the following people for their contribution to *Osteoporosis Prevention: A Proactive Approach to Strong Bones & Good Health.*

Jennie Cook, Sandy Coulter, Lisa Cox, Cathy Davis, Joel Figatner, MD, Andy Gero, Mary Hall, Monica Hang, Jane Hill, Dean Lange, Lois Lange, Mary McFarland, Mary Mercado, Jeannette Messerlian, Kay Moyer, Ed Newton, Marian Newton, Pam Philips, Irene Poff, Robert Poff, B. Burt Rahavi, MD, Carol Roope, Rowene Roseth, Sydney Rott, Debra Sawatsky, Roger Talish, John S. White, Kevin Williams, Charlene Wilson and the unmentioned participants. They have made valuable suggestions, corrections and comments regarding the portions of the book they examined. They are not responsible for any possible errors, nor do they necessarily endorse the material contained in this book.

The authors of the osteoporosis and densitometry books listed in the bibliography. They helped me obtain the technical background needed to write this book.

GE Healthcare, Juvent, Inc., and Skulls Unlimited International. Photos from them have been reproduced in this book.

Don Nelson, Bonnie Nelson, and Chivorn Chum. They've provided technical assistance.

Louise Harris Berlin. She has spent hours carefully editing *Osteoporosis Prevention*. Thanks to her, this book is much easier for laypeople to read and understand.

My sincere thanks to all of these contributors for their kindness and help.

Preface

I'm not a medical professional, which means I'm not able to give you personal medical advice, and **you should consult your doctor before doing anything mentioned in this book**. Nevertheless, this book can help you prevent osteoporosis and get top-quality care.

For example, my experiences with bone density testing can help you learn where you should be tested and what type of bone density reports you should be getting.

It's normal for readers to question my qualifications: I've spent two years researching osteoporosis and analyzing density reports. In addition, I've received help from physicians, nurses and physical therapists. I'm also able to write this book because:

◆ **I'm an author**. I've written eight consumer books on jewelry and gems, which have been sold worldwide.

◆ **I have more than fifteen years' experience translating technical material into everyday English**. As a result, I'm able to research medical texts and journals and understand them. The principles of physics and chemistry apply to a wide range of subjects, including both gemology and the study of bones. Bone, in fact, is a gem material.

◆ **I've spent a lot of time with people with broken bones**—my mother, my neighbors, and patients in the orthopedic department of a hospital where I volunteer. This has helped me understand their suffering.

◆ **I have experience writing about consumer issues** such as how to choose a jeweler and read a gem lab report. Therefore, it's easy for me to discuss topics like how to choose a bone-density test center, how to avoid being duped by testimonials and how to be a savvy patient.

◆ **I have several sets of my own bone density test results to share with you**. An in-depth case study of an individual can sometimes be just as revealing as a group study. Hopefully, you'll be better able to interpret the details of your reports if you study mine.

◆ **I don't have a financial interest in any of the products or services discussed in this book**. This helps me be more objective and open to all points of view.

What I Hope to Accomplish

All of my gem books promote education and consumer issues; this book does too. Specifically I wrote *Osteoporosis Prevention* in order to:

◆ **Help prevent osteoporosis.** Osteoporosis organizations and many medical professionals have the same goal; but as an author of gem and jewelry books, I can reach people they may miss. Getting the masses to take care of their bones is a challenge and will require a group effort.

◆ **Encourage people to be more proactive about their health care and to ask for copies of their test results.** We shouldn't expect doctors to be fully responsible for our health. We must educate ourselves.

◆ **Help patients get maximum benefit from their density reports.** Some doctors only use bone density reports as a means of diagnosing osteoporosis and monitoring the effects of drugs on the disease. Bone density tests can also help spot some back and alignment problems. In addition, they can help us design effective exercise programs that fit individual needs. Chapter 15 offers ideas on how to better use the results of your bone density tests.

◆ **Help medical professionals motivate patients.** Throughout this book, I relate how different events and test results have made me take action to maintain good health. Hopefully my experiences can help health care providers find ways to motivate patients and get them more involved in their health care.

◆ **Encourage bone density test centers to take a more active role in osteoporosis prevention.** A logical place for people to learn how to have strong bones is at a bone-density testing center. There is time during the test to answer patients' questions and to bring up topics such as nutrition and exercise. Yet many people I've interviewed have told me they've received no written or verbal information from their testing center on how to prevent osteoporosis or interpret their test results.

Some testing places provide this information, but I think all bone density centers should be taking an active role in osteoporosis prevention. This would enable patients who don't see a doctor during or after the test to get feedback and advice.

1

Why I Decided to Write a Book on Osteoporosis

In the summer of 2003, I got a surprise when I learned the results of my bone density test. I had low bone mass in my spine (osteopenia) and the bone density of my hip had gone down 7.3 percent in the past 2 ½ years.

Natural methods of preventing bone loss had not been sufficient. I'd eaten well-balanced meals, I'd never smoked, I'd never dieted, I didn't drink coffee, my calcium and vitamin D intake were sufficient, I got lots of exercise, and I wasn't on any medications. My healthy lifestyle had paid off because I had no other medical problems, and my bone density was not seriously low. However, the declining density levels still concerned me.

After studying the results of my bone density test further, my list of questions grew. I wanted to know:

◆ **Is there a natural way to build bones that works?** The advice I'd followed had not prevented bone loss.

◆ **What type of calcium is best?** Much of the information I'd read was contradictory.

◆ **What types of exercise are most beneficial?** Regular weight-bearing exercise such as walking, dancing and running had not prevented me from losing bone. However, I believe that my bone density would have been much lower, had I not engaged in these activities.

◆ **Why was I losing bone at different rates in my body?** My spine density had decreased only 2.9 percent whereas the density of my hip had gone down 7.3 percent.

◆ **Why did some of my bones have a high density and others a low density** compared to younger women? Why did parts even within my own spine have different densities?

To find answers to these questions, I've read books and articles on osteoporosis, interviewed a number of people, and analyzed density reports of friends and relatives as well as my own. This process helped me learn why general weight bearing exercise such as running was not sufficient for maintaining my hip and spine density: running didn't target these areas—it targeted my legs and ankles.

What is Osteoporosis?

The National Osteoporosis Foundation defines "osteoporosis" as a "disease in which bones become fragile and more likely to break." If it's not prevented or treated, it can progress painlessly until a bone breaks. Fractures most often occur in the spine, hip and wrist. (www.nof.org)

Osteo means "bone" and *porosis* means "porous." Osteoporosis is a different condition than osteoarthritis, which comes from three Greek words meaning bone, joint, and inflammation.

After I started exercising the weak areas of my hip and spine, their density improved. Strength training was most effective. It made me realize how weak my back and hip muscles were and why it's just as important to have a well-rounded exercise program as it is to have a well-rounded diet.

I also took Fosamax, a drug that helps stop bone loss, but that wasn't sufficient. During one nine-month period while I was on the drug and not exercising my back muscles much, my spine density decreased. It went back up when I started strength training. By the time I finished this book, the densities of my spine and hip had reached normal levels.

Curiously, the interval during which I took the least supplemental calcium was the period where I had the most bone gain. Consequently, I no longer think it matters much what type of calcium I take. In fact, I'm now more concerned about getting too much calcium from supplements.

I decided it would be worthwhile to share what I learned from my research because I saw a need to encourage consumers to learn more about osteoporosis and bone density testing. Being well-informed can motivate you to take preventive measures and help you select a competent testing center. It can also help you discuss the subject intelligently with your doctor(s) and profit more from your osteoporosis tests.

Why I Care More about My Bones than the Average Person

When my mother was 62, she slipped on a throw rug and broke her left hip. Even though she recovered and was able to live normally, her life was not the same afterwards. She had to give up her job as a nurse and go on disability. Her left hip bothered her throughout her life because of arthritis and the large metal pin that was put in during her hip operation. Twenty years later she got the pin removed to help alleviate the discomfort, but this involved another painful recovery.

At the age of 83, my mother tripped over a stool and fell while rushing to answer the phone. Both bones in her lower left leg were broken. After another long recovery, she had a bone density test, which showed she had osteoporosis.

My grandfather was 92 when he broke his hip getting out of a chair. Since my aunt and uncle were physically unable to care for him during the recovery, they had to put him in a nursing home. My grandfather was so upset about this that he refused to eat, walk or do therapy. Eventually, he died-indirectly of a broken hip. A neighbor of mine died for the same reason, but at a younger age.

One morning a week, I volunteer in the orthopedic-neurology ward of a local hospital and talk to the patients. This serves as a continuing reminder of what life is like when you break a bone, hurt your back or have joint problems.

I used to be an international tour director. This gave me the opportunity to see the brighter side of aging. Many retired people take advantage of their free time to travel abroad, and some of them are in their 80's and 90's. It was not unusual to see them participate in activities such as walking the Great Wall of China.

I recall one passenger, a 95-year-old man whom the group called "Pappy." Almost every night he would dance with women in the group. Even after a tiring flight from Bali, Indonesia to Sydney, Australia, Pappy was ready to go out dancing on the town. Meanwhile, the 30- and 40-year-old passengers just wanted to go to bed.

Another passenger, who was 88, told me he spent much of his free time mountain climbing and cross-country skiing. Some tour directors I met while traveling were in their 70's and 80's.

I've seen the enthusiasm and zest seniors can have for life. I know how witty and sharp their minds can be. Consequently, I look forward to life in my 80's and 90's, and you should too. However, for maximum enjoyment, it helps to have strong bones and good health. Throughout this book, you'll find preventive measures that can help you achieve this. They are summarized in Chapter 18, the last chapter of the book.

A variety of experiences have made me care more about my bones than the average person, but seeing my mother suffer with her broken hip and leg has probably had the greatest impact. I decided to write this book to help other people avoid what my mother went through.

Short Answers to Basic Questions about Osteoporosis

Below are some commonly-asked questions regarding osteoporosis. It will give you a quick overview of the subject and help you understand the basic concepts of the book. Afterwards, you may wish to read Chapter 18, "How to Help Prevent Osteoporosis and Broken Bones." This final chapter reviews the principles of osteoporosis prevention and helps make the rest of the book more understandable. Quizzes on the first five chapters also help reinforce fundamental points.

1. What is osteoporosis?

Osteoporosis is a disorder of the skeleton in which bones become fragile and susceptible to fractures. If it's not prevented or treated, it can progress painlessly until a bone breaks.

2. Who gets osteoporosis?

Anybody can get osteoporosis; but women are more likely to develop osteoporosis than men because their estrogen decreases at menopause, which often results in significant bone loss. However, men also get osteoporosis. People with a family history of osteoporosis or fragility fractures are more susceptible to getting osteoporosis. For more information, see Chapter 3, "Who is at Risk?"

3. What causes osteoporosis?

The most common causes of osteoporosis are inadequate diet, smoking, heavy drinking, insufficient weight-bearing activity, drugs such as corticosteroids, and a decrease in estrogen or testosterone. Certain diseases can also lead to osteoporosis. Chapter 3 lists diseases and drugs that can cause osteoporosis.

4. How is osteoporosis diagnosed?

Ultrasound and various types of x-rays are used to detect osteoporosis. The most common test for diagnosing osteoporosis is called a DXA test (dual energy x-ray absorptiometry). Chapter 14, "Bone Density Testing," describes the diagnostic methods in more detail.

5. What can I do to prevent osteoporosis?

　a. **Eat a balanced diet with adequate calcium, vitamin D and magnesium**. A heart-healthy diet, low in saturated and trans fats but high in fruits and vegetables, is ideal. Reducing fat calories will allow you to eat more bone-nutrient-rich foods without gaining weight, especially if the diet is combined with aerobic exercise.

Chapter 9, "Other Bone Nutrients," discusses a variety of vitamins and minerals that help maintain and build bone, and it lists the best food sources for them.

b. **Participate in weight-bearing activities** that include exercises targeting the hips, spine and wrists— three areas especially susceptible to fracture. Chapter 5 has a list of exercises, yoga poses and general activities that target these three areas.

c. **Take vitamin and mineral supplements if necessary**. Chapters 8 and 9 will help you determine if you're getting enough of the most important bone nutrients.

d. **Avoid smoking and excessive drinking**. They impair calcium absorption and inhibit the growth of bone-building cells.

e. **Do whatever is necessary to stay healthy.** A person's overall health affects their bones. In addition, the drugs needed to treat some diseases can lead to bone loss.

f. **Consider adding soy foods to your diet.** They contain plant estrogens, which may help reduce bone loss. See Chapter 9 for more information.

g. If the preceding measures aren't sufficient for maintaining adequate bone density, **consider taking preventive drugs**. Chapter 11 discusses the risks and benefits of osteoporosis drugs.

h. If your bone density is low, **find out about vibrating platform therapy when it becomes available in your area**. This involves standing for 10–20 minutes a day on a device that has barely perceptible vibrations, which stimulate your bones. It was introduced in Europe in the fall of 2005 and as of January 2006 was still undergoing research for approval by the FDA in America. See Chapter 12.

i. **Learn about bone density tests before being tested.** You'll profit more from the test results. They don't just tell you if you have osteoporosis or not. They can help you design an exercise program to strengthen areas of low bone density, and the images can reveal a variety of medical problems. See Chapters 13, 14, 15 and 17.

j. **If possible, select an information-oriented test center that provides detailed reports of the spine and hip.** Besides serving as a diagnostic tool, bone density reports can help you create an exercise program that is right for your needs.

6. How is osteoporosis treated?

Osteoporosis is treated with the above preventive measures and with drugs such as Actonel®, Boniva®, Didronel PMO®, Fosamax®, Evista®, calcitonin, Forteo®, Protelos® (strontium ranelate) and hormone replacement therapy. Braces are occasionally used to help support the spine, hip pads may be recommended to help prevent hip fractures, and surgical procedures may be used to treat vertebral fractures. Referrals to physical therapists may be provided; these specialists can recommend safe exercises and help patients improve their posture. Chapters 7 and 11 discuss drugs and posture.

7 How much calcium is recommended?

The recommended amount can vary from one country to another. In the US, the Institute of Medicine of the National Academy of Sciences recommends 1000 mg/day for adults 19 to 50 years, 1200 per day for adults over 50, and 1300 mg/day for children 9 to 18 years of age.

In Great Britain, the Scientific Advisory Commission on Nutrition recommends an intake above 700 mg/day in the normal population. It states that there is inconclusive evidence that more calcium may be needed, but further research is necessary. They recommend 1200 mg/day for adults diagnosed with osteoporosis (www.nos.org.uk).

8. How can a person determine the amount of calcium in their food?

In the US, you can just look for the Percent Daily Value on the food label under "Nutrition Facts." Since this value for calcium has been set at 1000 mg per day, you only need to drop the % sign from the Percent Daily Value for calcium and add a zero.

For example, on an American carton of milk, it typically states that in one cup of milk you get 30% of your Daily Value. This means one cup of the milk provides 300 mg of calcium. A cup of fortified orange juice or a slice of Swiss cheese can supply a similar amount. Chapter 8 lists the calcium content of a variety of foods.

9. Why not just take a calcium supplement instead of trying to get it from food?

It's best to try and get your calcium from food because you'll also get other important bone nutrients along with it. In addition, calcium from food is more natural and may be better absorbed than calcium from pills. One notable exception is spinach, which has a high amount of oxalates, substances that bind with calcium and prevent it from being absorbed. See Chapter 8 for more information on calcium and substances that may inhibit its absorption.

10 When should I have a bone density test?

If you're a woman, it can be helpful for you to establish a baseline for your bone density either at the age of 50 or around the time of menopause, whichever comes earlier, provided you get a detailed, written report. Even if the results are normal, you can use the information to design an appropriate exercise program for yourself in order to prevent osteoporosis. Establishing a baseline can also help you determine your rate and amount of loss during menopause. No matter what the results may be, examining your test results can increase your awareness of osteoporosis and encourage you to take preventive measures against it.

Men aged 70 or older should be tested. And whether you're a man or a woman, bone density tests are usually advisable if you:

◆ have had a fracture resulting from minor impact

◆ have a chronic disease that causes bone loss

◆ take antiseizure drugs or steroid type drugs such as prednisone and cortisone

◆ take high doses of thyroid medication

◆ have had a loss of sex hormones at an early age

11 What type of bone density test should I get?

A DXA (dual energy x-ray absorptiometry) test of the spine and hip. Chapter 14 discusses the various types of bone density tests.

12 Does a DXA bone density test involve a lot of radiation?

No. The radiation dose of a DXA bone density test is about 1/10 that of a chest x-ray and 1/500th of a CT scan. You'll get about as much radiation from a DXA test as you would during a transcontinental flight. One big advantage of a DXA test is that it can provide images of the skeleton using very low radiation. If a problem is noted, these can be followed up with regular x-rays, which are sharper and provide greater detail. Figures 1.1 and 1.2 are examples of DXA images.

13 What is osteopenia?

It's pre-osteoporosis; in other words it's the precursor of osteoporosis. *Penia* means "lack" or "deficiency." The term originated from the Greek goddess of poverty, Penia. A diagnosis of osteopenia means your bone density is lower than normal but not yet full osteoporosis, and it can encourage you to take steps to prevent further bone loss.

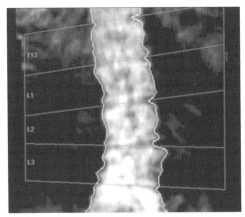 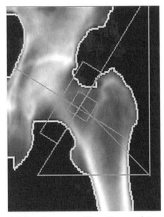

Figs 1.1 & 1.2 DXA images of a lumbar spine and hip. Images like these show visually the areas of highest density (the whiter the area the higher the density). They also give doctors clues about potential alignment or disc problems and in some cases indicate where fractures have occurred. *Photos from GE Healthcare.*

14 What is a T-score?

On a bone density report, a T-score is a statistical number that compares the bone density of an area of your skeleton to that of a normal, young adult. T-scores can vary from one skeletal area to another.

According to the guidelines of the World Health Organization, the worst score of the important skeletal areas should be used to establish a diagnosis of osteoporosis or osteopenia. Like the weakest link on a chain, the site with the lowest bone density is at highest risk of fracture. For a more in-depth discussion of T-scores, see Chapters 13 and 14, "Understanding Density Reports" and "Bone Density Testing."

15 Do all countries have the same definition of osteoporosis?

According to the World Health Organization (WHO), a T-score of -2.5 or lower indicates the presence of osteoporosis. Countries throughout the world have adopted this standard. However, densitometers can vary in the way they measure bone density and assign T-scores. This means it's important to be retested on the same densitometer to accurately compare your test results. Chapters 14 and 17 discuss issues regarding the accuracy and reproducibility of bone density tests, and they compare the results of two pairs of my tests done on different densitometers at about the same time.

2

Density Versus Strength

Which of the materials below is the most dense (compact)?
Which is the strongest (resistant to breakage and fracture)?

◆ Pure gold
◆ Diamond
◆ Jade
◆ Bone

If you think that gold has the greatest density, you're right. It's over five times more dense than diamond, the hardest and next most dense of the four substances. Yet pure gold is not any stronger than bone, the least dense of the four materials.

The strongest of the four is jade. Diamonds can chip or crack if you hit them just right, but jade resists breakage because of its internal structure of interlocking crystals. In fact, jade is so strong that ancient civilizations used it for axes and weapons.

The purpose of this little quiz is to illustrate that density and strength are two separate physical properties. **Bone density** refers to how tightly bone tissue is packed and to the amount of mineralized tissue in a given volume of bone. Even though there is usually a high correlation between bone density and bone strength, people with low bone mass can have strong bones, and people with good bone density can have bones that are susceptible to fracture. Unfortunately, bone density tests are not able to measure bone strength.

Susan Brown, PhD, director of the Osteoporosis Education Project in Syracuse New York, discusses this phenomenon in her book *Better Bones, Better Body* (pp. 42–44). People in Singapore and Hong Kong, for example, have a lot fewer hip fractures than Western populations even though their bone density is not any greater. Brown believes their healthier diets contribute to their stronger bones.

If you combine pure gold with other elements such as silver, copper and zinc, you can make it a lot stronger. The strength is largely determined by the quantities and types of elements used along with the gold. The strength of our bones is also largely determined by their composition. We need more elements than just calcium in our diet to form strong bones. That's why it's important to include lots of fruits and vegetables in our diet. They contain many elements not found in meat and processed food. Protein, however, is also important for bone strength. The basic structure of bone consists of a soft protein framework (mostly collagen), which hardens when calcium, phosphorous and other elements are deposited on it. (**Collagen** is a fibrous protein constituent that binds our skin, cartilage, bone and other connective tissue. The term is of Greek origin and means "glue producing.") The classic medical reference *Gray's Anatomy* states:

> That collagen contributes much to the mechanical strength is clearly demonstrated in bones treated to denature or remove their collagen, when the bone becomes brittle and fragile. . . . It is clear that besides contributing to the tensile, compressive and shearing strengths of bone, the small degree of elasticity shown by collagen imparts a measure of resilience to this tissue, helping to resist fracture when mechanically loaded (p 461, 38th edition).

Bone Health and Osteoporosis, a Report by the Surgeon General makes the same point in simpler English.

> Bone is a composite material, consisting of crystals of mineral bound to protein. This provides both strength and resilience so that the skeleton can absorb impact without breaking. A structure made only of mineral would be more brittle and break more easily. While a structure made only of protein would be soft and bend too easily (p 18).

A gold alloy (metal mixture) can be strengthened by working it with processes such as pressing, pulling and rolling. Similarly, we can increase the strength of our bones with weight training, resistance exercises, and impact activities such as tennis and running. Stretching can help make both our muscles and bones more flexible.

Gold can be porous (filled with little pits and holes) when it is improperly cast. Metal with holes in it is naturally weaker than smooth, dense metal. Likewise, the more porous bones become, the more likely they are to break. The term *osteoporosis* means porous bone.

One of the best ways to determine if you have osteoporosis is to have a bone density test done. Density tests are discussed in detail in Chapters 13–15 of this book. Keep in mind, however, that even though bone density is important, so is bone strength. When comparing osteoporosis drugs, you should consider how they affect fracture rates as well as bone density. To get maximum benefit from the drugs, you'll also need to get the proper nutrients and exercise for your bones.

Factors other than diet and exercise can affect bone strength and density. They are discussed in the next chapter.

Quiz: Chapters 1 & 2

True or False?

1. Bone density tests do not measure bone strength.
2. Calcium improves the flexibility of bones.
3. People with normal bone density can be susceptible to fractures.
4. When comparing osteoporosis drugs, you should consider their impact on fracture rates as well as bone density.
5. The hips, spine and wrists are especially susceptible to fracture.
6. Osteoarthritis usually precedes osteoporosis.
7. After menopause, women have no hope of restoring bone loss.
8. Men seldom get osteoporosis.
9. The World Health Organization has established guidelines for diagnosing osteoporosis, which are used worldwide.
10. Bone density testing is only beneficial for diagnosing osteoporosis and osteopenia.
11. If you have osteoporosis, you'll eventually break a bone.
12. One big advantage of a DXA bone density test is that it can provide images of the skeleton using very low radiation.

13. Osteoporosis means _____ _____ in Greek.
14. Osteopenia means _____ _____ in Greek
15. Name at least five common causes of osteoporosis.

16. Your bone density report says your results are normal. This means:
    a. You don't have to exercise.
    b. You are not at risk for fractures.
    c. You can eat a lot of junk food.
    d. None of the above
    e. All of the above

17. Your bone density report indicates you have osteopenia in the spine. This means:
    a. You should see an orthopedist.
    b. You might have a fractured vertebra.
    c. Your bone density in the spine is lower than normal but not low enough to be classified as osteoporosis.
    d. None of the above
    e. All of the above

Answers:

1. T Density and strength are separate physical properties.
2. F The calcium component of bones makes them hard and less flexible. Their collagen protein renders them more pliable and resilient.
3. T However, in most cases the higher your bone density, the lower your risk of fracture.
4. T
5. T
6. F They're separate diseases. Osteoarthritis affects the spaces between the bones, the joints.
7. F
8. F
9. T.
10. F Bone density tests can also help detect other medical problems. In addition, they can help you design an exercise program that fits your needs, provided that you get a detailed, written report.
11. F Many women with osteoporosis never break a bone. However, your chances of a fracture are much higher if you have osteoporosis. It's best to avoid fractures before they happen by taking preventive measures.
12. T
13. Porous bone
14. Bone deficiency, low bone mass, or any similar translation
15. Inadequate diet, smoking, heavy drinking, insufficient weight-bearing activity, a decrease in estrogen or testosterone, certain diseases, and drugs such as corticosteroids. The next chapter discusses the causes of osteoporosis in more detail.
16. d If you'd like to be healthy and have your bone density stay normal, get good nutrition and exercise. Normal bone density scores do not mean you are immune to fractures; you are simply at lower risk.
17. c A diagnosis of osteopenia is a warning sign. Use it to motivate you to take preventive action against osteoporosis. If you don't already do strength and resistance exercises, this is a good time to start.

3

Who is at Risk?

Anybody can get osteoporosis if they don't get adequate nutrition and exercise, or if they are taking bone-robbing medications. However, thin, postmenopausal women with a family history of osteoporosis are especially susceptible to the disease. The next two sections discuss these and other risk factors.

Osteoporosis Risk Factors You Cannot Change

Age
The older you are—male or female—the more likely you are to get osteoporosis. People normally reach peak bone mass sometime between the ages of 25 and 40. After that, bone density typically declines.

"Women have two phases of age-related bone loss—a rapid phase that begins at menopause and lasts 4-8 years, followed by a slower continuous phase that lasts throughout the rest of life." (pp 43 & 44 of *Bone Health and Osteoporosis: A Report of the Surgeon General*)

Children and young adults can also get osteoporosis, but their bone loss is often the result of inadequate diet, medication use or another medical condition, not their age.

Gender
Women develop osteoporosis more often than men, largely because their estrogen levels abruptly decline in mid life, and their bones initially tend to be thinner. However, men get osteoporosis too.

In his book *Beautiful Bones Without Hormones* (p 53), orthopedist Leon Root says, "One in eight men will develop osteoporosis in his lifetime, and after the age of seventy, the risk of developing this 'silent killer' is the same in men as it is in women." This bone loss can be caused by low levels of testosterone, which may partly result from excessive alcohol consumption or some prostate cancer treatments. Testosterone is also gradually lost as part of the aging process. A simple blood test can measure testosterone levels.

Race

Caucasian and Asian people are more apt to get osteoporosis than people of Hispanic or African heritage. However, people of any ethnic background can get osteoporosis.

Heredity

A family history of osteoporosis or bone fracture increases your risk of osteoporosis. In her book *The Osteoporosis Handbook* (p 20), Sydney Lou Bonnick, MD, says that medical studies of identical twins and of daughters of women with osteoporosis suggest that the amount of bone we are capable of making is largely determined by an inherited ability to make bone.

Body Type

If you are thin-boned, of low weight, and petite or tall, you are at greater risk of osteoporosis and fractures than people who weigh more and have thicker bones.

Menstrual History

You have a higher risk of osteoporosis if you began menstruating after the age of 16 or if you reach menopause before the age of 45, either naturally or surgically. The lower your exposure to estrogen over your lifetime, the higher your risk of osteoporosis.

Previous Fractures

If you've had a fracture resulting from a low-level trauma, you are more at risk for osteoporosis and another fracture than people who have never had a bone fracture.

Osteoporosis Risk Factors You Can Change

Diet

A diet low in Vitamin D and essential minerals such as calcium and magnesium increases your risk of osteoporosis. (See Chapters 8 and 9.)

A diet with excessive protein and excess salt is also a risk factor because it increases the loss of calcium in the urine (see pages 18 & 19 of *The Osteoporosis Handbook* and pages 123–128 of *Better Bones, Better Body* by Susan E. Brown, PhD). Nevertheless, you need protein to build bones. In essence, you should have a well-balanced diet.

Are You at Risk of Osteoporosis?

You might be at risk if you answer "yes" to one or more of the following questions. The more "yes" answers, the greater your risk.

1 Have you had a fracture resulting from minor impact?

2 Have your parents or siblings had osteoporosis?

3 Have your parents or siblings had fractures due to minor impact?

4 Do you have a history of cigarette smoking?

5 Are you a heavy drinker?

6 Have you had a height loss of more than an inch (3 cm)?

7 Are you thin, and do you weigh less than 127 pounds (58 kilos)?

8 Are you taking steroids or antiseizure drugs?

9 Do you have a very sedentary lifestyle?

10 (women) Have your periods stopped for more than 12 months?

Overdieting Excessive dieting can reduce a woman's estrogen levels and deprive the body of essential nutrients required for bone building. Osteoporosis is a common result of eating disorders such as anorexia and bulimia. Gastric surgery may also lead to osteoporosis.

Lack of Exercise An inactive lifestyle or prolonged bed rest can reduce your bone density. Exercise that makes your body work against gravity, resistance and/or weight is one of the most effective ways of maintaining strong bones. The most physically active children are typically the ones who reach the highest peak bone mass. See Chapter 5 for more information on how exercise can build bones.

Smoking The nicotine and cadmium found in cigarettes can have a direct toxic effect on bone cells. In addition, smoking robs your body of estrogen and lowers the amount of calcium absorbed from the intestine. Smoking is also associated with an earlier onset of menopause and a higher risk of fracture. (*The Osteoporosis Handbook* p 17 and *Bone Health & Osteoporosis: A Report by the Surgeon General*, pp 139 & 140)

Excessive Alcohol

Excess alcohol is toxic to osteoblasts, the cells that build bone; it can also damage the liver and pancreas, thereby affecting the body's ability to absorb calcium and make vitamin D. Chronic heavy drinking also lowers levels of estrogen and testosterone and may increase the likelihood of fracture.

Some studies suggest a moderate alcohol intake in women increases bone density, but it does not seem to lower fracture risk. (P. 140, *Bone Health & Osteoporosis: A Report by the Surgeon General*)

Excessive Caffeine

A high intake of caffeine increases the loss of calcium in the urine and thus the loss of bone. Miriam Nelson, PhD, author of *Strong Women Strong Bones,* states "caffeine consumption over about 400 milligrams per day—the equivalent of four cups of coffee—doubles the risk of hip fracture" (p 63). Besides having a diuretic effect, it often replaces liquids that contain calcium.

Diseases & Disorders that can Lead to Osteoporosis

The following diseases and types of disease may lead to osteoporosis by either reducing the absorption of essential nutrients or by affecting the cells that build or break down bone:

◆ Digestive diseases: Inflammatory bowel disease, celiac disease, Crohn's disease malabsorption,. Surgical removal of the stomach or parts of it can also increase your risk of osteoporosis.

◆ Chronic kidney disease

◆ Chronic liver disease

◆ Chronic lung disease

◆ Hyperthyroidism

◆ Hyperparathyroidism

◆ Cushing's syndrome

◆ Cancer

◆ Anorexia nervosa

◆ Rheumatoid arthritis

◆ Multiple sclerosis

◆ Endometriosis

◆ Female athlete triad. This is a combination of three interrelated conditions associated with intense athletic training—disordered eating, osteoporosis, and amenorrhea (absent or irregular periods). Exercise burns calories, so the more you exercise, the more you must eat to maintain normal body weight. For more information on the female athlete triad, see the website of the American Academy of Family Physicians: www.aafp.org or their June 1, 2000 issue of the *American Family Physician,* pp 3357-3364, which can be downloaded from their website.

If you have one of these diseases or conditions, you may wish to ask your doctor if it would be advisable to get a bone density test to determine the effect of the disease on your bones.

Medications that can Cause Osteoporosis

The medications listed below can increase your chance of osteoporosis. If you're taking any, discuss them with your doctor and ask if you should monitor your bone density.

◆ **Corticosteroids** (also called glucocorticoids or steroids) (e.g., cortisone, prednisone, dexamethasone). These are prescribed for conditions such as arthritis, asthma, lupus, and chronic lung disease. Steroids can lower blood levels of estrogen and testosterone and slow bone formation. According to the 2004 *Report of the Surgeon General* (p 46), corticosteroids are the most common cause of **secondary osteoporosis** (osteoporosis which is the byproduct of another condition or drug use).

◆ **Excessive thyroid medication** (e.g., Levothroid, Synthroid)

◆ **Antiseizure medications** (e.g., Dilantin, phenobarbital, Carbatrol, sodium valproate, diphenylhydantoin). When taken over a long period of time, they can interfere with calcium absorption and the production of vitamin D.

◆ **Diuretics** (e.g., Bumex, Edecrin, Lasix). Besides preventing fluid buildup by causing the kidneys to excrete water and sodium, they also cause the kidneys to excrete more calcium.

◆ **Chemotherapy**. It may prematurely shut down your production of estrogen, depending on the kind of chemotherapy and your age. Radiation can also affect bone density.

◆ **Hormone deprivation therapy** (used to lower the blood levels of male and female sex hormones, also called GnRH agonists). This medication is used to treat prostate cancer and endometriosis.

◆ **Long-term use of Heparin**, a blood thinner

◆ **Long-term use of Depo-Provera** for birth control

◆ **Antacids that contain aluminum**. The aluminum can interfere with calcium absorption if you take too much of the antacids.

    Never change the dose or stop taking the medication without first discussing this with your doctor.

For more information drugs and diseases that may cause bone loss, consult:

http://www.surgeongeneral.gov/library/bonehealth/factsheet4.htm

Better Bones, Better Body (pp 160–166 & 180–188) by Susan Brown, PhD

Bone Health & Osteoporosis: A Report by the Surgeon General, 2004, by the United States Public Health Service

The Osteoporosis Handbook (pp 20–24) by Sydney Lou Bonnick, MD

Quiz: Chapter 3

1. Which of the following is not a risk factor for osteoporosis?
   a. age
   b. gender
   c. menstrual history
   d. obesity
   e. heredity

2. Osteoporosis can result from the long-term use of
   a. vitamins e and c
   b. cholesterol medication
   c. cortisone and predisone
   d. none of the above
   e. all of the above

3. Osteoporosis can result from the long-term use of
   a. antiseizure medications
   b. high doses of thyroid medication
   c. steroids
   d. none of the above
   e. all of the above

4. Name at least four osteoporosis risk factors that people can control.

True or False?

5. Postmenopausal bone loss is caused by estrogen deficiency.

6. Osteoporosis in young adults is often the result of inadequate nutrition, another medical condition, or the use of certain medications.

7. If people get good nutrition and sufficient calcium, and they don't smoke or drink excessively, they won't get osteoporosis.

8. The older we get, the higher our risk of developing osteoporosis.

9. Men's bones are not affected by decreasing hormone levels.

10. You should consult your doctor before stopping medication or decreasing the dosage.

11. If neither your parents nor your grandparents had osteoporosis, you don't need to be concerned about preventing bone loss.

Answers:

1. d

2. c

3. e

4. Poor nutrition, insufficient exercise, smoking, excessive drinking, excessive caffeine, over dieting.

5. T

6. T

7. F Illness, medication, inactivity, and decreasing estrogen levels at menopause are four other factors that can lead to osteoporosis.

8. T

9. F Low levels of testosterone can lead to bone loss in men.

10. T

11. F Even if close relatives haven't had osteoporosis, you can still get it; but your risk is generally lower than that of someone with a family history of osteoporosis. It's possible that family members unknowingly had osteoporosis. It's only within the past twenty years or so that osteoporosis testing has been encouraged.

4

Basic Bone Terminology

The more you understand about your bone density tests, the more you'll benefit from them. Information from my density reports has been the prime factor in motivating me to take steps to strengthen my bones. If I see on paper comparative results that show my bone mass is decreasing, it's a much stronger incentive than just hearing generalized warnings about middle-aged women losing bone.

Thorough tests usually measure the density of your hip(s) and lower spine using some type of low-energy x-ray device. In order to understand the test results, you should know a little about the anatomy of these areas.

What is the Hip?

In strict medical terms, there is no hip bone. If someone breaks a hip, they have broken the top part of the **femur**, the upper leg bone. The femur, also called the thighbone, juts out at the top and then connects to the pelvis at a ball and socket joint called the hip joint.

The hip area of the femur is divided into three main areas called the head, femoral neck and trochanteric region (see figure 4.1) The two areas where most hip fractures occur are the:

Femoral neck   The narrow section of the upper femur located next to the ball-shaped end of the femur, the **head**. The density of the femoral neck is often used to predict the overall risk of body fractures.

Trochanteric region   The part of the femur just below the femoral neck. It includes two knob-like areas called greater trochanter and lesser trochanter, which aid the attachment of muscles between the thigh and pelvis. Often on density reports the trochanteric region is simply called the trochanter or troch.

Besides indicating the densities of the neck and trochanteric region, comprehensive bone density reports also state the density of your **total hip**, which also includes part of the leg bone below the trochanteric region, called the **shaft**.

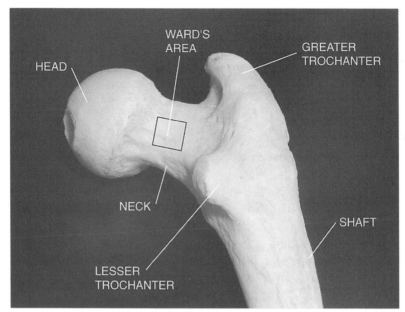

Fig. 4.1 Femoral hip. *Photo by Ed Newton.*

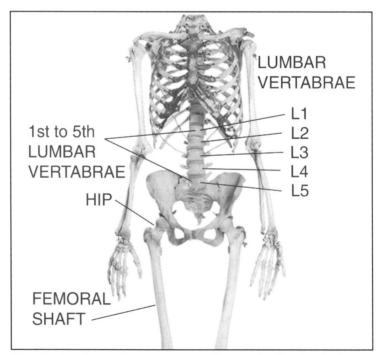

Fig. 4.2 Skeleton photo courtesy of www.skullsunlimited.com

Included on the report will be a small square area in the femoral neck called Ward's area or Ward's triangle (it's square on the image). It's an area of diminished density where the femoral neck is connected to the main shaft of the bone. The density results of this area are not normally used for diagnosing osteoporosis of the hip (p 251, *Bone Densitometry for Technologists* by Sydney Lou Bonnick). The primary areas of concern are the femoral neck, the trochanteric region and the total hip.

Spine Terms Found on Bone Density Reports

In most cases, spine density tests only measure the first four bones of the **lumbar** (lower) spine. These bones, called **lumbar vertebrae,** have an opening through which the spinal cord passes, and they are labeled from top to bottom as **L1, L2, L3, L4** (fig. 4.2). The L stands for "lumbus," which is the Greek word for "loin." The lumbar spine also has a fifth vertebra, L5, and in rare cases a sixth one, L6.

Depending on the density center and the density machine used, a variety of spine terms may be encountered. Some are defined below:

Lumbar spine   The part of the back between the lowest pair of ribs and the top of the pelvis. Since ribs don't hide the lumbar spine, it's practical to measure the density of this spine area.

                        On density reports, this term may refer to L1–L4, L2–L4 or another area determined by the radiologist. Check the report to see how the spine is defined.

AP spine: L1-L4   Another term for lumbar spine. Technically it means the x-ray beam passed through the top four lumbar vertebrae on an anterior to posterior path instead of a lateral path when the density was measured.

PA spine: L1–L4   Same as previous term, except the results are based on a posterior to anterior x-ray path.

Basic Bone Terms

If your doctor recommends medication and you wish to do some prior research on it before you take it, knowing a few bone-related terms will help you understand drug information leaflets and medical journal articles. Bone is composed of three types of tissue:

Bone marrow   A soft substance that fills the holes and passageways of the trabecular bone. It contains red and white blood cells.

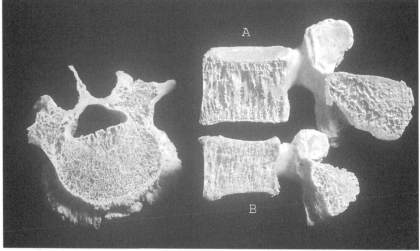

Fig. 4.3 Left: Cross section of a human vertebra showing the inner sponge-like trabecular bone and the outer more solid cortical bone. Right: two longitudinal views of human vertebrae. The upper vertebra (A) is less dense than the lower one (B).

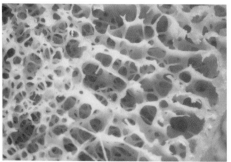

Fig. 4.4 Photo of a cross section of a vertebra taken through a gemstone microscope at 10x

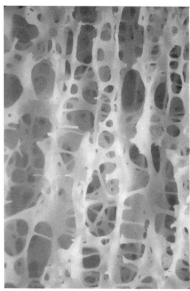

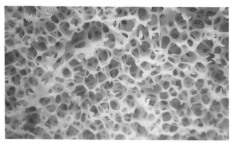

Fig. 4.6 Cross section of trabecular bone of higher density than that in figure 4.4 (10x)

Fig. 4.5 Longitudinal view of vertebral trabecular bone at 15x. The thicker and better connected the bone framework and the smaller the holes, the stronger the bone.

All photos this page by Renée Newman

Cortical bone   A dense outer layer of bone that is made of fibrous pro-
(compact bone) tein inlaid with deposits of minerals such as calcium,
                           phosphorous, magnesium and potassium. These minerals
                           mix with water to form a cement-like substance that
                           makes the bone strong and hard. The long bones of the
                           arms, legs and ribs are mostly cortical bone.

Trabecular   A porous inner layer of bone with a lattice structure that
bone   resembles a sponge. The vertebrae, pelvis, and small
                           bones of the wrist are composed mainly of trabecular
                           bone. The neck and trochanter region of the hips also
                           consist primarily of trabecular bone. The combination of
                           compact cortical bone with a supple core of spongy bone
                           is what makes bones both strong and light.

Bone is a living, self-regenerating tissue. Even though our body reaches its peak bone mass sometime between the ages of 25 and 40, new bone continues to form throughout our life while old bone is dissolved. The breakdown and removal of old bone is called **resorption**. The entire process of removing and building bone is termed **bone remodeling** or **bone turnover**. It is achieved with two types of bone cells:

Osteoclasts: Cells that dissolve and clear away old bone by secreting
                           an acid. This process releases minerals into the blood
                           and creates microscopic cavities on the bone surface.

Osteoblasts: Cells that build bone by filling in the cavities created by
                           the osteoclasts. Afterwards the osteoblasts are trans-
                           formed into mature bone cells that are alive but inactive.

Bone remodeling allows our bodies to repair damage caused by wear, and it helps our skeleton adapt to stress by forming new bone. In addition, it ensures that enough calcium and other minerals circulate in the blood to carry out the bodily functions that depend on these minerals.

My explanation of the above terms was based mainly on information in:

Beautiful Bones without Hormones, by Leon Root, MD, orthopedic surgeon
    at New York's Hospital for Special Surgery

Bone Densitometry for Technologists by Sydney Lou Bonnick, MD, medical director of the Clinical Research Center of North Texas and Lori Ann Lewis, MRT, CDT

Gray's Anatomy: The Anatomical Basis of Medicine and Surgery, Thirty Eighth Edition, Churchill Livingstone staff

Quiz: Chapter 4

Matching

_____ 1. Femur   a. Breakdown and removal of bone

_____ 2. Trabecular bone   b. Lower back

_____ 3. Cortical bone   c. Fourth lumbar vertebra

_____ 4. Lumbar region   d. Thighbone

_____ 5. Bone remodeling   e. Bone-eroding cells

_____ 6. Resorption   f. Bone-building cells

_____ 7. L4   g. Sponge-like inner bone

_____ 8. Osteoblasts   h. Compact outer layer of bone

_____ 9. Osteoclasts   i. Replacement of old bone with new bone

True or False

10. Bone density tests of the hip usually measure the upper part of the femur.
11. Spine density tests frequently measure the bone densities of the first four vertebrae of the lumbar spine.
12. The two areas of the hip where most fractures occur are the femoral neck and the trochanteric region.
13. The pelvis, femoral neck and the trochanteric region are three of the sites that are often measured on bone density tests of the hip.

Answers

1. d
2. g
3. h
4. b
5. I
6. a
7. c
8. f osteoBLasts BuiLd bone.
9. e osteoCLasts CLear away and erode bone
10. T
11. T
12. T
13. F The femoral neck and trochanteric region are often measured, but not the pelvis.

5

Making Exercise Safe **and** Fun

When I was in high school, running a mile in gym was something I dreaded. It exhausted me and sometimes I felt nauseated because my body wasn't properly conditioned. Today I look forward to running a mile in the morning. Instead of repeating laps around a track, I run down tree-lined streets viewing the sunrise and waving at passers-by.

My goal is to run a mile in less than ten minutes without feeling breathless, tired or sore afterwards. I've achieved this by *gradually* increasing the distance and running speed. It's safest to start exercising gradually with short, regular sessions. In addition, it's easier to find twenty minutes in the morning to walk, run and stretch than an hour.

How We Know that Exercise Makes Bones Denser

The easiest way to determine the effect of exercise on bone density is to compare the densities of people who exercise and people who don't. Numerous studies indicate that athletes have higher bone densities than non athletes. For example, an article in *Clinical Orthopedic and Related Research* (p 179-182, 1971) indicated the following results of a study of athletes and non athletes:

◆ All the athletes had a higher bone density than the non athletes.

◆ The non athletes who exercised had a higher bone density than the ones who didn't exercise.

◆ The bone density of the thighs of weight-lifters was the strongest, followed by runners and soccer players. The swimmers had the lowest bone density.

Just as muscles get stronger the more you use them, bones become stronger and denser when you place demands on them.

The effects of exercise can also be seen when comparing the densities of people before and after they are bedridden. Inactivity results in decreased bone density, muscle strength, and blood circulation. Consequently, patients are now encouraged to get up and walk soon after surgery.

We can also compare different bones in a person to determine the benefits of exercise. For example, x-rays and bone density tests of tennis players have shown that the playing arm has larger and denser bones than the other arm. The bone density can be much as 35% higher than the non-playing arm (J Bone Joint Surgery [Am] 1977, 59: 204–208).

What Types of Exercise are Good for Bones?

Two types of exercise important for building and maintaining bone mass are:

Weight-bearing exercise: This is any exercise in which your body is bearing your weight and working against gravity, e.g., walking, running, stair climbing, etc. Swimming, on the other hand, is not a weight-bearing activity. The water supports your weight.

The importance of gravity on bones is confirmed by studies of astronauts after space travel. Weightlessness causes them to lose bone. (*Osteoporosis Handbook* by Sydney Lou Bonnick, MD, p 72)

The bones most directly affected by weight-bearing exercise are the ones most likely to increase in density and mass. For example, the feet, ankle and leg bones benefit more from walking than the hips, spine and arms. However, if you did a hand stand and started transferring weight from one hand to another, your hands, wrists and arms would get the most bone-boosting benefit. This is stated more scientifically by Dr. Clinton Rubin, a professor at the State University of New York who has spent over twenty years researching how bone grows and heals. He says, "Bone adapts its structure to become denser and stronger or weaker depending on functional demands. Adaptation from exercise and mechanical stimuli is local, unlike pharmacologic intervention, which systemically bathes the entire skeleton (and all other tissues) with a drug."

Strength training and resistance exercises: These include weight lifting using free weights and resistance exercises using body weight, resistance bands, and variable weight machines. Resistance exercises involve pulling, pushing or lifting. When the muscles contract during these exercises, the tendons to which they're attached pull against the bone, stimulating bone cell activity and bone growth. The stronger the muscles, the more they stimulate the bones.

Comparative studies show that strength training is more effective at building bone than low impact exercise such as walking. Two of these studies are described on page 9 of *Strong Women, Strong Bones,* by Dr. Miriam E. Nelson, director of the Center for Physical Fitness at Tufts

University. In her research, Nelson found that walking had no effect on bone density in the hip, but there was a slight benefit to the spine. Strength training, on the other hand, helped postmenopausal women gain an average of one percent in a year, whereas the volunteers in the control group who didn't exercise lost about 2 percent of their bone density. In addition, the participants who strength-trained increased their scores on a balance test by 14 percent, further reducing their risk of fractures. (Published also in the 1994 *Journal of American Medical Association* 272: 1900-1914)

High impact activities such as running, basketball and vertical jumping can benefit bone more than walking, but they are also harder on the joints.

There are two other types of exercise that are important for people concerned about osteoporosis:

Back strengthening exercises: Exercises that gently arch the back or focus on good posture can strengthen the back muscles. This helps prevent a stooped posture, which puts stress on the spine and increases the risk of spinal fractures. Swimming also strengthens back muscles.

Balance exercises: These reduce the risk of falls and fractures. After the age of fifty, our sense of balance may gradually decrease. Standing on one leg, walking on the toes or with one foot directly in front of the other (tandem walk) are examples of exercises that improve balance.

My Experiences with Four Types of Exercise

Before starting any exercise program, you should consult your doctor. But even if he or she gives you a clean bill of health, exercise may do you more harm than good if you don't start slowly and do it properly. I've had positive and negative experiences with four kinds of exercise. My goal is to help you obtain the benefits but avoid the injuries that I've had.

Running: At the beginning of this chapter, I mentioned that, if I'm home, I run a mile almost every morning. When I run regularly, I have more stamina and endurance than when I don't, so I've always been motivated to continue. Running gives me more aerobic benefit than any other exercise I do.

Coaches and doctors often say that it's better for the joints to run on dirt, grass or asphalt than to run on cement. I used to run in parks and on the grassy areas between the street and the sidewalk. However, after tripping on hidden sprinklers or holes and spraining my knees and ankles a few times, I decided to run on residential streets facing potential traffic. Fortunately, I haven't tripped over anything since.

When I was about 35, I had a chiropractor who specialized in sports medicine check my running form. One thing he told me is that it's easier on the back to run fast and smooth than to run slow and bouncy. Therefore, I don't jog. Lately I've modified my running so that it's more like race walking than running because I place my heel down before my toe. That, too, is supposed to reduce stress on the back. In addition, it helps prevent tripping when the muscles are conditioned to raise the front part of the foot while placing the heel to the ground.

Over the years I've learned how to avoid pulled muscles and how to feel refreshed instead of tired after running. Here is what I do.

◆ I warm up by walking two or three blocks.

◆ If I ever feel a pain anywhere, I immediately stop running and just walk until the pain goes away, which it almost always does quickly.

◆ I never take pain medication, not even aspirin or Tylenol, because I want to know if and where I have pain in order to avoid reinjuring the affected area. I don't run with injured muscles.

◆ When I haven't run for more than a week, I start back gradually by alternately running a block or two and then walking. I do this until I feel I can run a continuous mile while breathing easily and talking at the same time. Later I work on speed.

◆ I stretch my calf and front and back thigh muscles after running. I used to do it before running until I pulled a muscle once.

◆ I wear shoes with proper cushioning that are designed for running.

For me, the key to safe running has been to do it gradually and regularly. Before a person can safely run, they have to be able to walk without getting breathless, tired or sore.

Yoga: I started attending yoga classes in the late 90's when a fitness center opened in my home community. I like yoga because it relaxes the mind, and it improves muscle flexibility, balance, breathing and strength.

During a yoga class in December 2003, I strained my back muscles. They got better, but two months later I strained them again doing yoga. Consequently, I stopped attending yoga classes.

Later at a book convention, I met a yoga instructor who told me he had ended up in a hospital with excruciating back pain after doing a pose in a yoga class. He said that some yoga poses should be avoided, depending on the student. He's learned what he shouldn't do, and he's had no problems with yoga since. He even teaches it.

At the same convention, I met another yoga enthusiast, whose wife teaches yoga. When I told him how I'd strained my muscles doing yoga, he said part of the problem could be that yoga classes at fitness centers are often too large for the teacher to verify if the poses are done correctly by everyone. For one thing, when doing a forward bend, the stomach should always be pulled in so that the stomach goes toward the spine and the back is flat.

A high percentage of the poses and exercises my yoga teachers chose involved bending over to touch the floor or the toes. In addition, the teachers sometimes had "focus on the back" sessions in which they also did a lot of western type exercises such as stomach curls and straight leg lifts while laying on the back. Perhaps the large number of back activities combined with the high amount of bending I'd been doing in my everyday activities was too much for my back muscles.

Several books I've read have advised people with osteoporosis to avoid forward bending exercises. In her book *Walk Tall*, Sara Meeks, a physical therapist specializing in osteoporosis, advises patients to:

> Watch out for exercises that can harm your back. If your current exercise program includes sit-ups, straight leg raises, toe touches or knee-to-chest movements, *you are at risk!* Research has shown that forward-bending (flexion) exercises can cause compression fractures of the spine [in people with osteoporosis].

I still do a few yoga poses at home. Some that involve placing body weight on the hands can be especially effective at strengthening the wrist, an area susceptible to breakage. Other poses help me maintain muscle flexibility better than other forms of exercise. Yoga is also excellent for improving balance and breathing.

A couple of my yoga teachers related how they had been in accidents and that yoga had been the only form of therapy that had been able to relieve their back problems. Yoga can be extremely beneficial provided it is done correctly.

Weight Training: The results of my 2004 bone density tests made me decide to sign up for weight and resistance lessons with a trainer. The day after my first thirty-minute lesson of upper body training, my arm muscles had hardly any strength left. By the third day my arms were so sore I could hardly use them to eat or wash my hair. Later I had burning sensations in the muscles so I stayed home and rested. A week later my arms started feeling normal again. My strong desire to improve the density of my spine and hip kept me from giving up the training.

I waited two weeks before resuming the weight training, but from then on, I did half the number of repetitions as before, and I had the trainer work both my upper and lower body so no one part would get overused in a session. Afterwards I didn't have any problems. After six months of weight training, I had my bone density retested. The density of both my spine and hips increased (See Chapter 15).

Weight training is one of the most effective ways to maintain and build bone. However, it can injure your muscles if done improperly. Here are a few guidelines to prevent injury:

◆ If you've never lifted weights or used resistance machines before, **have a certified trainer or physical therapist show you how**. Proper form with the right amount of weight is important, but this is hard to learn from a book. You should also learn how to adjust the resistance machines to suit your height and have the trainers verify that you can do the exercises correctly.

◆ **Don't assume that trainers know your limitations.** If you can do the exercises easily without straining, they may overestimate your ability. Tell them you want to **start out slowly** and work different parts of your body, not just one area in a lesson. Some of the books I read after my session suggested no more than eight reps per exercise the first time. For out-of-shape people, three reps may be the limit.

Dr. Joan Bassey, an advisor to the National Osteoporosis Society in the UK, suggests that fewer reps with heavier weights is the best way to increase bone mineral density (BMD). Her book, *Exercise for Strong Bones,* coauthored by exercise practitioner Susie Dinan says on page 86:

> Weight training can be practiced using small weights and many lifts; this is good for endurance but it does not improve BMD. To improve BMD you need to lift heavier weights quite slowly, a few times. It is important to work up to the heavier weights over several months so you do not injure yourself. Injuries, if they occur, are usually the result of 'too much, too soon' or poor technique.

In the Spring 2005 "Osteoporosis Report," the National Osteoporosis Foundation advises:

> Select weights so the muscle being trained becomes fatigued after 10 to 15 repetitions.
>
> Add weight as the muscles strengthen, but don't add more than 10 percent per week.

◆ **Warm up** with other exercise before strength training. The trainer at the fitness center suggested ten minutes on the aerobic exercise machines.

◆ **Breathe regularly**, instead of holding your breath during the exercises. Exhale with effort or exhale as you lift.

◆ **Make sure you do the exercise with good form**. Don't slouch as you fatigue.

◆ **Give yourself at least 48 hours between strength training sessions.** The longer and more strenuous the session, the more recovery time is required. Rest can be just as important as the exercises.

Fitness Machines: Until recently, I never used fitness machines because I considered them a boring means of exercise. I'd rather run on the street past changing scenery than on a treadmill. The only reason I joined a fitness club was to attend their yoga classes.

After noticing that the bone density of the neck of my hip was going down, I decided to add some aerobic exercise that targeted this area more than running. I tried out various machines at the fitness center such as the elliptical cross trainers and reclining bikes. At first I could only be on each one for about three minutes before muscles in my thighs and buttocks got tired, so I knew the machine exercise was working different muscles than running and walking.

A month before I started using these machines, a business associate told me that she had injured her knee on an exercise machine and required physical therapy. I now understand how new users might hurt their knees if they don't start gradually. Just after I progressed to staying on an elliptical machine for ten minutes, the back my knees felt tight and strange. After using a reclining bicycle another day for just eight minutes, I could hardly walk downstairs without my knees bothering me.

In other words, even people who are physically fit must start new types of exercise slowly in order to avoid muscle injuries. My heart had no problem adapting to the machines, but it took me about two weeks to a month before my muscles felt normal after using the machines for more than twenty minutes.

I've continued using the fitness machines because I've seen that they work different muscles than my other forms of exercise. Strong muscles can help protect bones from breakage during falls. If a bone does break, recovery is faster when the surrounding muscles are in shape. In addition, the fitness machines help increase endurance and allow you to better monitor your fitness level and progress.

Bone-Loading Activities for the Hip, Spine and Wrist

Earlier in the chapter, I mentioned that the bone density of the playing arm of tennis players is consistently higher than that of the other arm. That's because the density of bones can increase when they are subjected to impact, weight-bearing activities, gravitational pull, and mechanical force. Listed below are examples of activities that can help maintain or improve the bone density of three areas susceptible to fracture—the hip, spine and wrist.

Check with your doctor first before doing these activities. In order to prevent injury, have a qualified person show you how to use exercise machines and make sure that you can do the exercises with proper form before trying to use the machines on your own. It's even advisable to have a professional show you how to do general exercises correctly and check your posture. You can injure your knees, for example, if you do squats improperly or if your body is not conditioned for them.

You must progress gradually. One physical therapist, Carol Roope, says that a common mistake is for individuals to try and progress too rapidly with exercises that are either too advanced, use too many repetitions, or require too much weight. **Exercises should not be painful** at the time and you shouldn't hurt that evening or the next day. Some people minimize their pain with the hope that the cliché "no pain no gain" is true. Taking that approach can cause injuries and chronic problems.

If you're diagnosed with osteoporosis, ask your doctor for a referral to a physical therapist who can show you which exercises are safest and best for you. The therapist should preferably have specialized training in dealing with patients with osteoporosis. Therapists face a paradox—the type of bone-loading activity required to maximize bone gain may also be the type of activity most likely to cause a vertebral fracture. Depending on your bone densities and symptoms, a physical therapist can determine which level of activities is good for you.

Besides targeting areas susceptible to fracture, you should exercise the entire body and do stretching and aerobic activities.

Some bone loading activities for the hip

General exercises

Lunges (To avoid knee injuries, the knees should not extend past the toes.)
Squats (Lower positions work the hips more, but the knees should not
    extend past the toes.)
Single leg lifts (sides, front and back)
Step-ups that bring the knee up to hip level

Exercises using resistance machines or weights
Hip adductor and abductor machines
Single leg lifts (side, front and back)
Squats (The knees should not extend past the toes.)
Lunges (The knees should not extend past the toes.)
Hip flexors (bringing knees up above the waist)
Leg extensions
Leg press, dependent on how low you go and where you place your feet
Elliptical machines when in an uphill position (This is considered aerobic exercise, not strength training.)

Yoga poses
Warrior pose (*Virabhadrasana*)
Chair, thunderbolt or powerful pose (*Utkatasana*)
Extended side angle pose (*Utthita Parsvakonasana*)

General activities
Stair climbing (Two stairs at a time is more likely to work the hips; one stair at a time targets the muscles near the knees.)
Hiking uphill and downhill
Marching, bringing the knees up to hip level
Gardening while squatting and not bending over with the back
Lifting boxes with proper form—using your lower body, not your back
Squatting to play with children or pets
Standing from a seated position without using an arm chair to push up

Some bone-loading activities for the spine

Exercises using resistance machines and free weights
Lat pull-downs
Long pulley row, keeping the back straight and not bending forward
Cable machine rows, high and low, keeping back straight
Pull-ups
Back extensions
Rear deltoids
Shoulder press

General exercises and yoga poses
   There are many types of exercises and poses that can strengthen the back muscles and help maintain bone mass and improve posture, but it's questionable as to which general exercises and yoga poses will increase the density of the spine.

Activities
Lifting boxes with proper form
Rowing a boat, keeping back straight and not bending forward from waist

Some bone-loading activities for the wrist

General exercises
Wall and floor pushups
Wrist presses

Exercises using variable resistance weight machines and free weights
Wrist curls
Arm curls
Shoulder press
Triceps extensions

Yoga poses
Downward facing dog pose, (*Adho Mukha Svanasana*)
Upward facing dog (*Urdhva Mukha Svanasana*)
Plank pose (*Dandosana*)
Side plank or Side inclined plane (*Vasisthasana*)
Half moon (*Ardha Chandrasana*)
Crow or crane pose (*Bakasana*)

Activities
Grocery shopping (holding cans, bottles and bags)
Serving plates of food
Loading and unloading the dishwasher
Kneading bread
Shoveling snow
Volleyball
Rowing a boat with the back straight and not bending over from the waist
Carrying suitcases
Playing a musical instrument that you hold unsupported
Holding a pet while standing
Waxing a car using your hands and a cloth
Scrubbing pots and pans
Pushing a lawn mower
Because I'm not a doctor, physical therapist, trainer or yoga teacher, I haven't described these exercises in detail. For more detailed information, please consult the books of four specialists in osteoporosis-related exercise.
◆ *Exercise for Strong Bones* by Joan Bassey PhD & Susan Dinan
◆ *The Osteoporosis Handbook* by Sydney Lou Bonnick, MD, FACP

◆ *Strong Women, Strong Bones* by Miriam Nelson, PhD
◆ *Walk Tall: An Exercise Program for the Prevention & Treatment of Osteoporosis,* by Sara Meeks, PT, GCS.

Choosing a Trainer

Ask the following questions when selecting a trainer:

"What are your educational credentials as a trainer?"

Look for a trainer that has been certified. Some trainers only know how to use the machines. Certified trainers and those with a degree in physical education or kinesiology have studied human anatomy and know which exercises are best for the various parts of the body. Many fitness clubs won't hire trainers unless they know CPR and are certified or have a related university degree.

"What type of experience do you have as a trainer?"

Teaching skills and athletic experience are just as important as education.

"Have you ever trained people of my age, fitness level or injury history?"

It's helpful if the answer is yes, but not essential. Some trainers have never had clients above the age of 40 and may not realize the limitations of older people. Make sure you tell the trainer of any previous injuries. For example, I told my trainers that I'd injured my lower back muscles doing yoga and I wanted to make sure that I didn't hurt them again. Two of my trainers had undergone therapy for back injuries of their own and were able to use their experiences to help me avoid back problems.

One of the easiest ways of finding a trainer is to ask for recommendations at a health club or gym. Many centers offer training sessions and may let you do a sample lesson for free. I took advantage of this type of offer. Since I liked the trainer, I signed up for lessons. Because of schedule changes and limitations on availability, I ended up having four different trainers during the course of a year. I enjoyed the variety, and I benefitted from their diverse backgrounds by learning different tips and exercises from each of them. Two were physical education teachers, one was a coach and another had been a competitive weight lifter.

Seeing the consistencies among them was also enlightening. I told all of the trainers that I especially wanted to work on my hips and mid and upper back. For my hips, all of them recommended the hip adduction/abduction machines, squats and different types of single leg lifts. For my back they all had me use various resistance machines including high and low machine rows and the lat pull-down. They also had me do other exercises targeting my wrists and working my total body. None of them suggested that I do jumping exercises or some extra running and walking to increase bone density in the hip and spine. Even though jumping exercises can help build bone, they can be hard on the joints and spine. Avoiding the need for hip and knee replacements should be a concern.

For me, the training has paid off. My bone density increased, my muscles are far stronger, I have greater endurance and better posture, and my resistance to muscle injuries has improved—in fact I've had none since I started weight training.

If you're not in good physical shape and you want to work with a trainer at a gym, discuss this with the gym's fitness director. Ask him or her to assign you a trainer that suits your needs and level of fitness. Tell the trainer your goals too and discuss any previous injuries. If you've had a bone density test, indicate your areas of weakness. That way they can better help you achieve your goals. If you don't have money for a trainer, read the next section, and consider putting training lessons on your wish list when family and friends ask for gift ideas.

Making Exercise Fun

At the beginning of this chapter, I mentioned that I've made running more enjoyable by doing it outdoors past changing scenery instead of around a track or on a treadmill.

Exercise can be even more fun if you do it with others. There are, of course, group activities such as sports and dancing, But there are also many group exercise classes and hikes available for people of all ages, and they are often free of charge or low-priced. Try contacting the following places and organizations for information about exercise classes and hikes:

◆ **Senior citizen centers.** These are usually listed under Senior Citizens' Services and Organizations in the yellow pages of your phone book. You can also look them up on the Internet. Sometimes they are listed on the website of your local city.

◆ **Department of Parks and Recreation**. Even if they don't offer exercise classes, they may be able to tell you who does. Many small parks in my area have groups doing all types of exercise in the morning such as Tai Chi and Qigong as well as western calisthenics. They're free and the groups often welcome anyone as a participant.

◆ **Shopping malls:** Many malls open their doors early in the morning to let people take daily walks inside. A few even offer free exercise classes that may be led by medical professionals. They may require that your doctor fill out a form saying it is safe for you to participate.

◆ **Environmental groups such as the Sierra Club.** They often sponsor free hikes for different fitness levels and ages. When I moved to Southern California I went on some of the Sierra Club hikes and found it a great way to meet friends and learn about local hiking trails and recreational areas.

◆ **Retirement centers.** A few centers offer exercise classes and invite non-residents to attend free of charge. Some are even led by physical therapists or other medical professionals. Members can offer each other support and encouragement. Your doctor may have to fill out a form to say it's safe for you to attend.

◆ **Senior Care Centers at hospitals.** A few hospitals offer aqua-therapy or other types of classes at a nominal charge. Even if they don't, they may be able to refer you to a place that does.

◆ **Physical therapy centers.** Occasionally these places let seniors use their equipment for a nominal charge and give them a little guidance. If they don't, they may be able to refer you to exercise classes in your town.

◆ **The YMCA and YWCA**

◆ **Fitness centers:** You typically have to pay a monthly member charge to attend classes at the center, but the cost is relatively low. Even though people of all ages attend the classes, they are usually geared to young people who are physically fit. Beginner classes may also be available.

◆ **Yoga centers.** They normally charge a fee for their classes, which are often smaller than those at fitness centers. Various levels of classes are offered.

◆ **Osteoporosis organizations.** For example, an exercise program called Osteofit has been established by the Osteoporosis Society of Canada (B.C. division) and the Osteoporosis Program of British Columbia Women's Hospital and Health Centre Osteofit classes are small, or have two instructors, and are designed specifically for people with osteoporosis. British Columbia residents can call (604) 875-2555 for an information line and locations.

Ask your doctor and bone density center if they know of similar programs in your area.

Incorporating Exercise Into Your Daily Activities

Finding time to exercise is a challenge. However, even if you have a busy schedule, it's usually possible to do two or three hours of exercise a day simply by including exercise as a part of your everyday activities. Here are a few ways to make exercise a part of your daily life.

◆ **Do exercises when you watch TV or listen to music.** This is a perfect opportunity to kill two birds with one stone. Watching television does not have to be a sedentary activity. Exercises are more fun when you do them to music or do them as a dance.

◆ **Take the stairs instead of waiting for elevators.** It's often faster to walk up a flight or two of stairs than to wait for an elevator. Not only do you save time, you get good exercise.

◆ **Instead of driving, walk whenever possible**, and don't waste time trying to find the closest parking place when it would be faster to park further away and walk.

◆ **Choose recreational activities that involve exercise;** for example, hiking, swimming, biking, gardening, dancing, sports and shopping.

◆ **Stand up and walk when you read and think**. If you can't read and walk at the same time, then stand with your back and head next to a door or wall, and practice having good posture while you are reading.

◆ **When you're waiting in line, use the time to do balance and posture exercises.** Instead of wishing the line would move faster, tuck in your stomach and buttocks, pull your shoulders back, stand tall with head over shoulders and practice balancing your weight on one leg at a time.

◆ **Choose volunteer activities that involve exercise.** For example, I know hospital volunteers who specifically select assignments that involve wheeling patients, delivering flowers, and running errands throughout the hospital. Four hours on duty can equate to an hour or two of exercise.

Some people train for walkathons to raise money for charity, some build houses for the disadvantaged, others help with children's sports. There are many volunteer activities that can help you remain in good physical shape while helping others at the same time.

How to Help Seniors Maintain their Muscles & Bones

It's possible to maintain your muscles and bones without ever setting foot in a gym. For example, a nurse told me how her grandmother in the Philippines lived to be 91 without ever breaking a bone or having to go to the hospital.

Her grandmother, who had had ten children, never drove; she always walked. To avoid having to go to the grocery store so often, she grew her own food and had farm animals. In the morning and afternoon, she fed the chickens. She also ate lots of fish, frequently with the bones in them. She was always happy and in a good mood. Up until the time she passed away with pneumonia, she lived normally in her own home, and she always had a straight back.

This grandmother was probably in better physical shape than many teenagers, simply because she engaged in a variety of activities throughout the day. In America, seniors often go to retirement or assisted living centers where all the daily chores are done for them. As a result they miss out on opportunities to use their muscles in normal everyday activities such as cooking, gardening, cleaning, doing the laundry, playing with children and taking care of pets.

Even when seniors remain in their own home, they or their children hire caregivers who often feel that they should wait on the elderly and do all the household chores since they are getting paid. The best caregivers, however, are the ones who help seniors do things for themselves, yet provide companionship. I know from experience.

For twelve years after my mother had a stroke, I was involved in her care, even though I lived out of town. Thanks to excellent therapists, she was able to recuperate enough to go back to her own home and get around with a walker. Here are some things I learned that can help the elderly maintain the use of their muscles:

◆ **Let seniors get out of the car and out of chairs by themselves** instead of rushing to help them. They need to practice using their muscles to get to a standing position without assistance. However, exceptions should naturally be made if they are sick or unable to walk.

  Placing a cushion on a chair or seat may give them the extra boost they need to try getting up by themselves. Making sure that chairs being used are non-slip and have arms will also encourage independence. In addition, this can help seniors sit down slowly with control instead of falling into the chair.

◆ **Take seniors to the grocery store and let them do their own shopping**. Just accompany them and help them carry the grocery bags. It's a good strength-training exercise for the hands and arms to take cans and boxes from the shelves and place them in a grocery cart, and it's normally more fun for them than doing exercises with hand weights.

One therapist suggested that I have my mother push the grocery cart with her walker in it. But he added that I should probably wear a big T-shirt with a message saying "we are doing therapy," in order to avoid dirty looks from onlookers.

When elderly people have low endurance, it's helpful to bring along a folding stool, which can be placed in the shopping cart. This allows them to stop and sit for awhile. Chairs in stores are sometimes nonexistent or else placed far away.

Even though it's faster to buy groceries for older people by yourself, it's not as helpful as taking them to the store. Shopping is a diversion for them and an opportunity to walk and use their muscles.

◆ **Let seniors do as much for themselves as possible**. If they can walk and they're not sick and they want, for example, a glass of water or a snack, let them get it themselves, instead of waiting on them. They need to get up and walk.

◆ **Encourage seniors to cook for themselves and for family events.** You'll enjoy the benefits of some good homemade food, and this will make them feel useful. My mom made the best pancakes I've ever had. Despite the fact that she had arthritis in her hands and couldn't stand without holding onto something, she still was able to prepare them by herself for family events. Stirring batter, and flipping pancakes is good exercise for the hands and it helps the mind think constructive thoughts. If necessary, seniors can pace themselves and sit occasionally while preparing the food.

◆ **Encourage seniors to participate in household chores,** instead of having a housekeeper do everything for them. This can be hard if there's hired help, but sometimes circumstances may make this possible.

For example, my mother's caregiver had to go out of town for a week because of an emergency. During that time, my mother had to get her own food, wash the dishes, take care of her dog and be on her own. I was concerned until I visited her and saw how much more self-motivated she had become. For a while afterwards, she washed and put away the dishes herself. During that time she could move her arthritic fingers more easily. When she stopped using her hands for housework, they became more stiff, and she even had a hard time taking cards and letters out of envelopes.

Getting seniors to do chores can sometimes be a challenge, but it's worth it. It adds purpose to their life, keeps them active, and allows them to be contributing members of the household.

◆ **Encourage seniors to volunteer.** This allows them to use their minds and keep active in a meaningful way. Museums, churches, schools, charity organizations, animal shelters are some places that often need volunteers. To find opportunities in your community, search the Internet by typing in your city on a search engine and the word "volunteering." You can also do a search at www.volunteermatch.org. Just type in your postal code and select your area of interest. There are many benefits to volunteering. The next chapter gives a few examples.

◆ **Help seniors find transportation, if you can't drive them yourself.** Seniors need a social life outside of their homes, but when they're unable to drive or walk to public transport, they tend to become homebound and sedentary because they don't like to bother people and ask for rides.

People are quick to criticize the elderly for driving, but they're not as quick to help them find alternate transportation. Some communities offer good affordable transportation designed for seniors, but many don't. Or if they do have a transport system, the rides must be arranged a week or two in advance, and then the person may have to wait an hour to be picked up.

One of the best gifts you can give an older person is to help them maintain their independence. To do that, try and encourage them to gradually help themselves and be active.

Quiz: Chapter 5

Multiple Choice

1. Which activity is most effective for maintaining bone density in the hips?
   a. Walking
   b. Marching with the knees high
   c. Swimming
   d. They're all equally effective.

2. Which activity would be most effective for maintaining the bone density of the wrist?
   a. Writing a letter
   b. Brushing your teeth
   c. Putting cans and bottles in a grocery cart
   d. Sewing a dress

3. Which professional is most likely to have the strongest bones, assuming none of them smokes and all get equally good nutrition?
   a. A waiter or waitress
   b. A secretary
   c. A bus driver
   d. A bank teller

4. Which professional receives more training in prescribing exercise for medical problems?
   a. An internist
   b. A certified trainer
   c. A general practitioner
   d. A physical therapist
   e. An orthodontist

5. Resistance-machine exercises are more effective than walking for increasing spine density because:
   a. They can specifically target the back muscles, whereas walking targets the legs and ankles more.
   b. Resistance machines allow you to progressively increase the stress level of the exercise and continually challenge the bones.
   c. Resistance machines can generate more force on the spine than walking.
   d. All of the above
   e. None of the above. Walking is just as effective as resistance machine exercises at increasing bone strength and density.

True or False?

6. People with severe osteoporosis should avoid physical activity in order to prevent vertebral fractures and falls.

7. Total inactivity can lead to severe bone loss, even if you get enough calcium and good nutrition.

8. Weight-bearing activities are those that involve lifting weights.

9. Exercise helps you avoid fractures by helping improve your balance

10. If you take medication for osteoporosis, you don't need to exercise.

11. Deep forward bending can increase the risk of vertebral fractures in people with osteoporosis.

12. To maintain bones, you must be active for the rest of your life.

13. Exercises should hurt a little while you're doing them, otherwise they aren't doing any good.

14. Any physical activity is better than none, but weight bearing and resistance exercises are the best for building bone.

Answers:

1. b Walking and swimming are excellent forms of exercise, but walking does not target the hip muscles as much bringing the knees up to hip level while marching. Weight bearing activities stimulate bone more than swimming. Single leg lifts and exercises on hip abductor/adductor machines may be even more effective than marching for preventing bone loss in the hip.

2. c Lifting cans and bottles, which are like weights, stresses the bone more than sewing, writing and brushing your teeth.

3. a. Waitressing involves more weight bearing and resistance exercise than the other occupations. Lifting trays and plates is similar to lifting weights. Walking to tables stresses the leg and ankle bones more than standing at a bank teller window. But standing stresses them more than sitting.

4. d Physical therapists are specifically trained to prescribe exercises after a medical diagnosis is made by a doctor.

5. d

6. F Physical activity is essential for all people, but people with osteoporosis may have to limit their activities. That's one reason why it's best to start osteoporosis prevention early.

7. T

8. F Weight bearing activities are those in which the body has to remain upright against the pull of gravity. Lifting weights is usually categorized as a resistance-type exercise.

9. T

10. F To maintain bone and muscle strength, you must keep active and exercise. Osteoporosis drugs are most effective when you combine them with exercise and good nutrition.

11. T

12. T

13. F Don't ignore pain that occurs during exercise; it's your body's way of telling you that something is wrong, e.g., you've over exerted yourself, you've pulled a muscle, you're doing an exercise wrong, you're having a heart attack, etc. Exercise does not have to be painful to be beneficial. In fact in some cases, it helps alleviate pain from arthritis and other conditions. After surgery, it's normal to experience pain during and after therapy, but that's a different situation in which you are working with a trained physical therapist.

14. T

6

Why I Volunteer in an Orthopedic Ward

Retired seniors aren't the only people who volunteer; full-time workers like me also like to fit it into their schedules. The sense of satisfaction you get when you volunteer is good for your mental health, and the physical activities that may be involved are good for your muscles and your bones.

Why I Became a Volunteer

My mother had to retire from nursing as the result of a broken hip. In the ensuing years, she volunteered at three different hospitals. During one of my visits, she needed a ride to a volunteer meeting; so I accompanied her. I was impressed with what I saw and decided I'd like to become part of an organization with such wonderful, caring people.

A few months later, my mother broke her leg while hurrying to answer the phone. I wasn't familiar with the hospital environment and felt if I knew more about went on there, I'd be better able to help family members the next time an emergency arose.

Not long thereafter, I signed up at a hospital in my community for their volunteer orientation. Since I prefer to work with patients instead of at a desk, I requested to work in the orthopedic ward, the hospital area for patients with bone, muscle, and cartilage problems (e.g., bone fractures, torn ligaments, herniated disks, osteoarthritis, vertebral compression fractures due to osteoporosis). I transport patients, talk to them, help with meals, run errands for the nurses and bring the patients whatever they may need such as water, snacks, ice packs, reading material and blankets.

I continue to volunteer at the hospital because it makes me feel good when I can help people. In addition, I like the people I work with, and I look forward to seeing them each week.

Some Unexpected Benefits

I knew beforehand that I'd get a sense of satisfaction from volunteering, but there were other benefits I hadn't thought of, such as:

◆ **I've become more safety-conscious.** When you see patients in casts or with back injuries after falling off ladders, you understand the importance of using sturdy ladders and spotters. Likewise after you've talked to patients who have fallen down stairs, you start to use handrails more frequently and you try to avoid carrying items with two hands when going up and down stairs. In turn, this prevents falls and broken bones.

◆ **I'm more aware of the seriousness of infection.** I didn't realize that people could end up in the hospital for weeks just because of a little cut, puncture or insect bite. But after seeing a variety of such cases, I know I must take signs of infection seriously.

   For example, one weekend when I was visiting my mother, she showed me an infected toenail. Instead of waiting until Monday to get her to the doctor, I took her to the emergency room, which turned out to be the right thing to do. The toe was worse than we thought and the nail had to be taken off.

◆ **It's given me a broader perspective on bone health.** Fractures are not the only bone-related problems we may face as we get older. Every week I see patients with joint and back problems, many of which are caused by long-term wear and tear. When selecting an osteoporosis exercise program, we must be just as concerned about protecting our joints and our backs as we are about strengthening our bones.

◆ **I've received lots of free professional advice when talking to patients in the hospital.** Lawyers have given me legal advice; computer experts have provided technical suggestions; one photographer gave me good tips on lighting; scientists have given me information for my books. I've learned a lot while visiting with patients.

◆ **I'm more appreciative of my health.** When I see the immense suffering some people go though, my problems seem insignificant.

◆ **It's expanded my view of the world** because I have opportunities to spend time with people outside of my profession and circle of friends and family. This makes life more interesting.

Charity doesn't have to be restricted to money and gifts. Your time can be equally valuable. It doesn't matter what you do as a volunteer. Just select activities that you enjoy and that best utilize your skills and talents. You'll probably end up receiving more than you give.

7

Posture **and** Osteoporosis

Is Osteoporosis the Only Cause of Hunched Backs?

In most cases, poor postural habits are the cause of hunched backs. You can have a hunched back yet have a spine with normal bone density. On the other hand, you can have osteoporosis yet have a straight back. For example, soldiers, models and entertainers who have been trained to stand straight often have good posture, even if they get osteoporosis.

The root cause of poor postural habits is sometimes low self-esteem. A psychologist told me that patients with a poor image of themselves often display their insecurity outwardly with a hunched posture; this can occur regardless of age or gender.

In some cases, osteoporosis leads to compression fractures of the vertebrae in the spine, which in turn can cause a curvature of the back. When fractured, a vertebra can shatter and fall in on itself. The fractures may occur spontaneously or with activities as minor as opening a window, vacuuming or sneezing. If there is an uneven compression of the vertebral bone, it can form a wedge shape that thrusts the spine forward over itself. This can cause what is called "**dowager's hump**," an outward curvature of the upper spine, technically identified as "**thoracic kyphosis**." When the curvature is extreme, chest capacity diminishes and the abdomen may protrude, impairing breathing and digestion. There is a loss of height and pain may be intense, although the fracture may also go unnoticed. This condition is not just restricted to women. Men can also have it.

Osteoporosis medication is often prescribed to stop or prevent compression fractures. In some cases, these medications even help reduce the pain. Braces to support the spine are occasionally recommended. Spine fractures are also being treated with new techniques such as vertebroplasty and kyphoplasty, in which a bone cement is injected into the fractured vertebra. These procedures help stop the pain and in some case, partially expand the collapsed vertebra.

Compression fractures and poor postural habits are the direct causes of hunched backs. However, osteoporosis can lead to compression fractures.

Therefore it's important to treat it early, before fractures occur. If you do and you practice good posture, you can usually avoid having a hunched back.

How Easy is it to have Good Posture?

Speaking from experience, it's not at all easy to maintain good posture if you've spent years slouching while seated and standing. Most people aren't aware of their posture until someone points it out. Exercise can help improve posture, but the improvement is usually temporary.

I used to attend yoga classes regularly, and posture exercises were often included. For about a half an hour after class, I had good posture. Then I gradually returned to my habit of hunching over. I started paying more attention to my posture while working on this book and examining my bone density reports.

If you want to have good posture, you can; but you must have a strong desire and commitment to do whatever is necessary to avoid slouching. To keep yourself motivated to improve your posture, think of the benefits. Good posture:

◆ **Makes you look better**. When I took a portrait photography course several years ago, the teacher told us that one of the most important things we could do to make our subjects look their best was to tell them to stand up straight without being stiff. A quick change in posture would make a world of difference in their appearance.

◆ **Helps prevent backaches and fatigue** because it allows your muscles and joints to move more efficiently. However, just after you start trying to correct your posture, your back and stomach muscles may be a little sore because they're not used to the new positions. You can help alleviate the soreness by *gradually* changing how long you maintain good posture.

◆ **Helps you avoid muscle injuries**, especially when you combine proper posture with good body mechanics.

◆ **Improves breathing** because it expands the capacity of your chest.

◆ **Makes you feel better**. Picture in your mind the way depressed people stand. It's hard to imagine them with good posture. Then visualize happy, vibrant people. Chances are, you'll envision them standing up straight instead of slouching. Posture has an effect on your mental state.

◆ **Helps you keep your balance**, thus preventing falls and broken bones.

Below, I've listed many of the steps I've had to take to improve my posture. It's better now, but I still haven't reached the point where I automatically have good posture without thinking about it.

Tips for Having a Youthful Posture

It's a good idea to have a professional evaluate your posture. For example, ask a physical therapist, trainer, doctor, or chiropractor to watch you when you stand, walk and sit. They see things that you may be unable to see in yourself. If you don't have contact with a professional, ask a family member or friend to make comments.

To feel what it's like to have proper posture, stand next to a wall or door with your head, shoulders and rear touching it. Here are some characteristics of a good standing posture:

◆ Head over shoulders

◆ Chin and stomach tucked in

◆ Shoulders back, down and relaxed

◆ Chest held high

◆ Maintain arch in lower back

◆ Hips level with equal weight on each side of your body

◆ Knees straight but not locked

◆ Feet hip width apart with your weight evenly distributed on them

If you practice this position several times a day, you'll gradually get used to the feel of standing straight. Instead of taking time out of your schedule to practice this posture, you can also read the mail, magazines and newspaper standing next to a wall.

You can also read seated on a stool next to a door or wall. You may wish to place a rolled towel in the small of your back near your waist for lumbar support. Try to have your shoulders maintain contact with the wall.

Some other tips for improving your posture include:

◆ **Lie on your back when you sleep instead of curling up on your side.** This helps bring your shoulders back. If your shoulders are hunched forward for six to eight hours a night, it's harder to hold them back naturally when you're awake. To ease strain on your back, put a pillow under your knees.

   People who stand straight naturally can lie on their sides without it having a negative effect on their posture. However, people who slouch tend to reinforce their bad habits at night if they lie on their side.

◆ **Look at yourself in the mirror when you're nude.** Compare how youthful your body looks when you stand with good posture to how it looks when you slump. This should help motivate you to pull your shoulders back and stand tall.

◆ **Watch TV and relax in chairs with straight backs or that are designed to support your back** instead of in soft, cushy chairs. The more you slouch in chairs, the harder it is to stand with good posture.

.◆ **When you're at home, wear tight fitting clothes that show your curves.** They make you more aware of your posture than loose baggy clothes, especially if you look at yourself in a mirror.

◆ **Ask a family member or friend to tell you to stand up straight** when they see you slump.

◆ **Use a chair with a headrest** if you have a tendency to jut your head out when you work at a computer or read. This is a common problem with women, as they get older. However, placing your head against the headrest counters the tendency to throw your head forward, thus preventing neck and postural problems.

◆ **Wear flat shoes with good support as often as possible**. Shoe inserts that help you place your weight evenly on your feet can help align your body and improve posture.

◆ **Do strength-training exercises** for your back and shoulders as well as the rest of your body. They'll make it a lot easier to hold your body erect. Having a trainer who constantly reminds you of good form is an added bonus.

◆ **Take posture rest breaks when working,** especially if you're in a forward bent position during activities such as gardening. Throw your shoulders back, tighten your stomach and buttocks, and then relax. If you do this throughout the day, your posture muscles will get stronger.

◆ **Whenever you walk or work out on exercise machines, try to focus on your posture and stand as tall as possible**. This will help maintain your height and a straight back.

It takes time to train your body muscles and bones to slump. Likewise, it takes time to retrain your body to have good posture. However, the effort pays off. You'll end up being healthier and looking younger.

8
Calcium

A t the age of 94, Mikimoto, the founder of the cultured pearl industry stated, "I owe my fine health and long life to the two pearls I have swallowed every morning of my life since I was twenty." Pearls are primarily composed of calcium carbonate. Considering all the benefits of calcium, there may be some truth to Mikimoto's claim. Calcium is used throughout the body for:

◆ Heart function
◆ Muscle contraction and growth
◆ Blood clotting
◆ Various hormone functions
◆ General metabolism
◆ Building bone and slowing bone loss. This doesn't necessarily mean, however, that the bone density of adults can be increased just with calcium supplements. As the National Osteoporosis Foundation states: "A high calcium intake will not protect a person against bone loss caused by estrogen deficiency, physical inactivity, smoking, alcohol abuse or various medical disorders or treatments." (www.nof.org)

Calcium does not act alone. Other nutrients are required for it to be effective, some of which are discussed in the next chapter. The following sections provide guidelines for getting the proper amount of calcium.

How Do We Know That Calcium Helps Bone Growth?

Calcium is a major component of bone. Therefore it's logical that calcium is required for bone growth.

Several studies have shown the importance of calcium for building and maintaining bone. For example, one study at the University of Indiana compared the bone densities of 22 sets of identical twin children. Both twins received about the same dietary intake of calcium but one was given a calcium supplement. The twin that took the supplement developed a high-er bone density. (*The Osteoporosis Handbook* by Sydney Bonnick, p. 26)

In another study, the rates of hip fracture in two regions of the former country of Yugoslavia were compared during a six-year period by tracking hospital records. The district with the fewest hip fractures was a dairy region where the people averaged 900 mg (milligrams) of calcium per day. The other area grew more grains and vegetables and had an average intake of about 400 mg per person per day. Even though the population was similar, it had more than double the number of fractures of the dairy region. (American Journal of Clinical Nutrition, 1979, Volume 32, p 540-549)

How Much Calcium Do People Need?

The US National Institutes of Health (NIH) recommend that adults get **at least 1000 mg of calcium per day.** For adolescents 9–18 years of age, it recommends 1300 mg; and for adults aged 51+ it recommends 1200 mg **including calcium from food**. Older people require more calcium because they absorb less than younger adults. You can find these recommendations at the NIH website: www.ods.od.nih.gov/factsheets/calcium.asp#h3.

The above guidelines are based upon calcium from the diet and any calcium taken in supplemental form. For example, a senior citizen would satisfy his 1200-mg daily requirement of calcium if he gets 600 mg from milk products, 300 mg from dark green vegetables, 350 mg from a glass of fortified orange juice. The preferred source of calcium is through foods rich in calcium. If you get enough from food, you don't need a calcium supplement.

Many other countries have different recommendations for calcium intake. In Great Britain, for example, the Government Committee on the Medical Aspects of Food and Nutrition Policy (COMA) has set the recommended nutrient intake of calcium for adults at 700 mg per day. The UK National Osteoporosis Society, states that adults who have been diagnosed with osteoporosis may need to boost their calcium levels to 1200 mg per day. (www.nos.org.uk)

A World Health Organization report states that there is strong evidence that the requirements for calcium might vary from culture to culture because of dietary, genetic, lifestyle and geographic reasons. For example, societies that consume more animal protein need more calcium. (Source: www.who.int/dietphysicalactivity/publications/trs916/en/gsfao_osteo.pdf)

How to Determine the Calcium Content of Food

In the United States, one way to determine calcium content is to look for the Percent Daily Value on the food label under "Nutrition Facts." Since this value for calcium has been set at 1000 mg per day, you only need to drop the % sign from the Percent Daily Value for calcium and add a zero.

For example, if you look at the nutrition information on a milk bottle, it may say that a serving has 30% of the Daily Value. This means that one serving (one cup) has 300 mg of calcium. (30% of 1000).

For foods like fresh vegetables, which don't have labels, you can check the National Nutrient Database for calcium on the website of the United States Department of Agriculture. It's found at: www.nal.usda.gov/fnic/foodcomp/Data/SR14/wtrank/sr14a301.pdf

An easier way to get less detailed information about the calcium content of various foods is to look at the charts below. They have been compiled from information on USDA National Nutrient Database for Standard Reference. Dairy products, dark green vegetables, certain fish eaten with the bones, and calcium-fortified cereals and juices have the most calcium. Meat and fruits generally have low amounts of calcium, but they contain other nutrients essential for strong bones and good health.

Calcium content of one cup (237 ml) of dairy products in milligrams

Milk product	mg	Milk product	mg
milk:, canned, condensed, sweetened	869	milk:, canned, evaporated, nonfat,	742
ricotta cheese, skim	669	ricotta cheese, whole milk	509
yogurt, fat-free, plain	415	yogurt, fruit, low-fat	245–384
fat-free milk	302	whole milk	291
eggnog	330	hot chocolate	301
buttermilk	285	hot fudge sundae	207
milk shake, chocolate	188	low-fat ice cream, vanilla	184
yogurt, fat-free frozen	200	cottage cheese	156

Source: US Department of Agriculture Nutrient Database

Calcium content in milligrams of 1 ounce (28 grams) of cheese

Food	mg	Food	mg
Swiss cheese	272	provolone cheese	214
mozzarella, part skim	207	cheddar cheese	204
Muenster cheese	203	American cheese	163
blue cheese	150	mozzarella, whole milk	147
feta cheese	140	Colby, low-fat	118

Source: US Department of Agriculture Nutrient Database

Calcium content of one cup (237 ml) vegetables in milligrams

Vegetable	mg	Vegetable	mg
frozen collards, boiled	357	frozen spinach, boiled*	277
frozen turnip greens, boiled	249	spinach, boiled*	247
collards, boiled	226	turnip greens, boiled	197
frozen kale, boiled	179	frozen okra, boiled	177
bok choy, boiled	158	okra, boiled	101
artichoke, boiled	76	broccoli, boiled	72
tomatoes, canned	72	celery boiled	63
carrot juice, canned	57	Brussels sprouts	56
cole slaw	54	squash boiled	49
celery, raw	48	green peas, frozen, boiled	48
cabbage boiled	47	onions boiled	46
asparagus, boiled	41	carrots boiled	41
tomato sauce, canned	34	turnips, boiled	34
sweet potato, boiled	33	carrots, raw	30
spinach, raw	30	romaine lettuce	20
one baked potato with skin	20	cauliflower, boiled	20

green peppers, boiled	12	boiled potato, no skin, one cup	11
corn, canned, 1 cup	11	iceberg lettuce	10
tomatoes raw	9	butterhead lettuce	2

Source: US Department of Agriculture Nutrient Database

*Most of the calcium in spinach is unavailable to the body because of its high content of oxalic acid.

Calcium content of one cup (227 g) beans in milligrams

Type of Beans	mg	Type of Beans	mg
soybeans, green, cooked	261	white beans, canned	191
soybeans, mature, cooked	175	canned pork & beans	142
navy beans	127	green snap beans, boiled	82
pinto beans, boiled	82	garbanzo beans, canned	77
kidney beans, canned	61	kidney beans, boiled	50
black beans	46	canned green beans	35

Source: US Department of Agriculture Nutrient Database

Calcium content in milligrams of 3 ounces (85 grams) of fish or meat

Food	mg	Food	mg
sardines with bones	325	salmon with bones, canned	181
ocean perch	116	rainbow trout	73
lobster	52	halibut	51
crab, blue, cooked	50	shrimp, canned	50
catfish	37	pork loin, lean	25
lamb, lean	17	turkey, light meat	16
chicken, dark meat	15	chicken, light meat	13
tuna, canned	11	lean beef	9
salmon, without bone	6	ham	6

Source: US Department of Agriculture Nutrient Database

Calcium content in milligrams of miscellaneous foods

Food	mg	Food	mg
fortified orange juice 1 cup	350	frozen rhubarb, cooked 1 cup	348
Total cereal 3/4 cup	258	Pizza slice	250+
soy milk (calcium-fortified) 1 c	245	raisin bran, General Mills 1c	238
Boston clam chowder 1 cup	186	tofu, soft, one piece	133
fast food hamburger, single patty with condiments and bun	126	mineral water 1 cup (varies depending on brand)	5– 70
almonds 1 oz, 28 grams	70	chili con carne	67
figs, dried 2	55	dates one cup	57
blackberries 1 cup	46	hard-boiled egg one	25
wheat bread 1 slice	26	rye bread 1 slice	29

Source: US Department of Agriculture Nutrient Database

Calcium content in milligrams of some desserts and sweets

Food	mg	Food	mg
chocolate pudding 1 cup	306	pumpkin pie, 1 slice	146
molasses, blackstrap, 1tbsp	172	white cake, 1 slice	96
milk chocolate bar with almonds, 1.45 oz, 41 grams	92	coconut custard pie, 1 slice	84
eclair, one	63	chocolate cake 1 slice	57

Source: US Department of Agriculture Nutrient Database

What Type of Calcium Supplement is Best?

Calcium carbonate is the most common form of calcium supplement on the market, probably because it is the lowest priced. It contains more elemental calcium (about 40 percent) than other calcium compounds. One calcium carbonate pill may contain as much as 500 mg of calcium. Most of the major brands of calcium are composed of calcium carbonate. They are best taken with meals because they require gastric acid for absorption.

Calcium citrate, another calcium compound, is becoming more widely used. The Calcium Fact Sheet of The Office of Dietary Supplements states that calcium citrate is more easily absorbed than calcium carbonate in individuals with decreased stomach acid. Orthopedist Dr. Leon Root explains that calcium citrate has the advantage of containing acid, and this helps with absorption. As a result, calcium citrate can be taken with or without food (*Beautiful Bones without Hormones*, p 93 and p 97).

The maximum amount of calcium in a calcium citrate tablet is normally 250 mg because it has less elemental calcium (20–25 percent). If the back of the calcium citrate bottle says it has 500 mg of calcium per serving, then check the serving size, which will probably be two tablets.

The following table summarizes the advantages and disadvantages of calcium carbonate and calcium citrate.

Comparison of Calcium Carbonate and Calcium Citrate

Calcium Carbonate	Calcium Citrate
Usually lower priced	Usually higher priced
Is best absorbed when taken with food	Can be absorbed with or without food because it contains acid
Usually more calcium per tablet	Lower concentration of calcium
May cause gas or constipation	Normally no side effects

Other types of calcium supplements, which may be found in health food stores or vitamin specialty shops are:

Calcium phosphate. This calcium compound occurs naturally in milk and dairy products. When sold as a supplement in the form of dibasic or tribasic calcium phosphate, it has 30–39 percent elemental calcium.

Dr. Miriam Nelson, associate professor of nutrition at Tufts University, suggests people avoid supplements made from calcium phosphate because most women get plenty of phosphorus from their diet—and an excess can interfere with calcium metabolism (*Strong Women Strong Bones, p. 113).*

Calcium lactate. This dissolves more reliably than calcium carbonate. However, you have to take more tablets to get the same amount of calcium because it contains only about 18% elemental calcium.

Calcium gluconate. It has only 9% calcium, but is more soluble than calcium carbonate. Calcium gluconate usually costs more than calcium citrate and calcium carbonate.

The preceding compounds are sometimes added to food, so you may be getting them without knowing it. The labels indicate which type of calcium has been added. It might be good to get a variety of types of calcium.

If the food you eat in a day contains 1200 mg of calcium, you probably don't need to take a calcium supplement—you're already getting enough in your diet.

Substances that Reduce Calcium Absorption

Some substances can interfere with the body's ability to absorb calcium. These include:

◆ **Oxalates**. They bind with calcium and prevent it from being well absorbed. They're in foods such as spinach, collard greens, rhubarb, sweet potatoes, beet greens, almonds and beans. The calcium in spinach and rhubarb is almost completely unavailable to the body.

Oxalic Acid Content of Selected Vegetables

Vegetable	g/100g	Vegetable	g/100g
parsley	1.70	chives	1.48
spinach	.97	beet leaves	.61
carrot	.50	radish	.48
collards	.45	beans, snap	.36
Brussels sprouts	.36	lettuce	.33
sweet potato	.24	celery	.19
turnip greens	.05	kale	.02

Source: US Department of Agriculture Nutrient Database

◆ **Phytates**. They bind with calcium, too, and are found in whole grain breads, beans, nuts, seeds, and grains. The calcium in beans and peas is only half as available as the calcium in milk. You can reduce the phytate level in beans by soaking them for several hours in water, discarding the water and then cooking them in fresh water.

Oxalates and phytates only affect the calcium of the plants in which they're found, not the calcium found in other foods eaten at the same time.

◆ **Fiber**. Fiber, especially from wheat bran, hampers calcium absorption because of its phytate content. It's a good idea to eat wheat bran products an hour or two before calcium-rich foods. The fiber in fruits, vegetables and common cereals does not significantly affect calcium absorption. People with low calcium intake should be particularly concerned about the effect of fiber on the absorption of calcium. The average American tends to consume much less fiber per day than the level needed to affect calcium absorption. The benefits of fiber outweigh its potential negative effect on calcium.

◆ **Alcohol**. It can reduce intestinal absorption of calcium. In addition, it can inhibit enzymes in the liver that help convert vitamin D to its active form, which in turn reduces calcium absorption. However, the amount of alcohol required to affect calcium absorption is unknown. Evidence is conflicting whether moderate alcohol consumption is helpful or harmful to bone.

The information in this section is from the Office of Dietary Supplements and from the National Osteoporosis Foundation websites:

www.ods.od.nih.gov/factsheets/calcium.asp

www.nof.org/prevention/strategies_calcium.htm

Substances that Cause Calcium Loss

Some substances can cause calcium to be excreted in urine, feces and sweat:

◆ **Sodium**. Dietary sodium like sodium chloride (salt) usually increases calcium excretion. Other sodium compounds found in food include: sodium caseinate, monosodium glutamate, trisodium phosphate, sodium ascorbate, sodium bicarbonate, and sodium stearoyl lactylate.

◆ **Protein**. As protein intake increases, calcium excretion also goes up. However if a high protein and high sodium food also contains an optimal amount of calcium, this may help counteract the loss of calcium.

◆ **Caffeine**. It can temporarily increase calcium excretion and modestly decrease calcium absorption. This can be offset by consuming more calcium. One cup of brewed coffee causes only a loss of 2–3 mg, which is easily offset by adding a tablespoon of milk. Moderate caffeine consumption (one or two cups of coffee or tea per day) has little to no negative effects on the bones of young women who have an adequate intake of calcium.

◆ **Aluminum and magnesium antacids**. These can both increase urinary calcium excretion.

In essence, the more caffeine, sodium, protein and antacids you consume, the more calcium your body needs.

(Source: Office of Dietary Supplements of the National Institutes of Health: www.ods.od.nih.gov/factsheets/calcium.asp)

Guidelines for Consuming and Buying Calcium

◆ **Eat calcium-rich foods throughout the day** instead of only at one meal in order to maximize calcium availability for your bones. The body doesn't produce calcium by itself.

◆ **Take no more than 500 milligrams of calcium at one time.** Calcium is better absorbed when taken in smaller doses several times a day. In addition it's best not to overload your body with calcium. Excess quantities of calcium can cause a variety of degenerative diseases (see *Calcium Hypothesis of Aging and Dementia*, Volume 747 of the *Annals of the New York Academy of Sciences*).

◆ **Take calcium carbonate with meals** to improve absorption. Taking calcium carbonate with orange or grapefruit juice also boosts absorption because acid is needed for calcium absorption, be it from the stomach, citrus juice, or citrate. Calcium citrate can be taken on an empty stomach because it contains its own acid source.

◆ **Read supplement labels carefully** so you'll know how much calcium you're taking. Labels typically state the milligram amount per serving, but the serving size varies depending on the manufacturer and type of calcium. For example, the serving size of calcium citrate is often two tablets for 500 milligrams of calcium, because each pill only contains 250 milligrams. Some manufacturers even have serving sizes of four tablets. This makes it appear as if each pill has more nutrients than it actually has. When comparing prices, also note the type of calcium in the pill. Calcium citrate costs more than calcium carbonate.

◆ **Avoid calcium from unrefined oyster shell, bone meal or dolomite without the USP (U.S. Pharmacopeia) label**, as these historically have contained higher levels of lead or other toxic metals. This advice comes from the National Osteoporosis Foundation. The USP label indicates the ingredients of the brand have been tested for safety and match the label description.

You can test how well a capsule will absorb in your body by placing it in a glass of vinegar or warm water for about thirty minutes. If it hasn't dissolved within that time, it probably won't dissolve in your stomach. Milk is one of the most absorbable sources of calcium.

Consequences of Too Much Calcium

The National Osteoporosis Society of Great Britain states on their website "It is recommended that you do not exceed more than 2000-2500 mg of calcium a day. Exceeding the upper limit of 2000– 2500 mg calcium could lead to medical problems including milk-alkali syndrome (a high level of calcium in the blood) and may interfere with the absorption of other minerals" (http://www.nos.org.uk).

According to the US National Institutes of Health, 2500 mg per day is the upper limit for children and adults ages 1 year and older. Those limits include calcium from food sources as well as supplements.

Excess calcium isn't all excreted when it's not absorbed by the bones, some of it may be deposited elsewhere such as the joints, kidneys and blood vessels, where it can be detrimental. **Excess** calcium may cause the following problems:

◆ Arteriosclerosis (calcium deposits on the inside of the artery walls and consequent hardening of the arteries)
◆ Calcification of the aorta
◆ Arthritis
◆ Kidney stones
◆ Muscle cramps
◆ Fibromyalgia (non-specific muscle pain)
◆ Soft tissue calcification
◆ Brittle bones
◆ Dementia

These conditions are more likely to occur when the proportion of magnesium is too low to that of calcium. (Sources: *Users's Guide to Calcium & Magnesium*, pp 15 & 16 by Nan Fuchs, PhD, *Better Bones, Better Body*, p 248, by Susan Brown, PhD, *Calcium Hypothesis of Aging and Dementia*, Volume 747 The *Annals of the New York Academy of Sciences*). See the next chapter for more information on magnesium.

Excess calcium can occur when people consume a lot of food and beverages fortified with calcium and then take calcium supplements. For example, if during a day you consumed a glass of fortified orange juice, fortified breakfast cereal with milk, yogurt, tofu, cheese pizza, almonds and ice-cream, you'd be getting more than enough calcium, much of it in the form of additives (even most of the calcium in tofu is usually added). If in addition to all this dietary calcium, you took 1200 mg of calcium pills, you'd probably be getting excess calcium. Calcium supplements are unne-cessary and possibly detrimental when you get enough calcium from food.

One of the problems in the preceding scenario is that there probably would not be enough magnesium in the diet to offset the excess calcium, unless you also took a magnesium supplement. When calcium is added to foods, manufacturers seldom add sufficient magnesium along with it, and more often than not no magnesium is added. Health problems are more likely to occur when there is a severe imbalance of minerals in the diet. See the next chapter for more information on magnesium and other nutrients needed for healthy bones.

If you take multivitamins, calcium tablets, and or consume calcium-fortified nutritional drinks and fortified foods, check the labels to see how much calcium you are getting. You might be getting too much. As mentioned earlier, the advice to get 1000–1200 mg of calcium a day *includes* the amount of calcium you get in food. It does not mean you should get an additional 1200 mg of calcium per day from supplements.

I've included several calcium-content tables in this chapter in order to help you determine if you're obtaining enough calcium from food, which is the best way to get calcium. On some days, it may not be possible to consume enough calcium in food and beverages. On those days, it's appropriate to take a calcium supplement. However, try to avoid using pills as a substitute for calcium-rich foods. Food not only supplies you with the calcium, it also provides you with many other nutrients required for strong bones and good health.

Is Coral Calcium Better than Other Calcium?

Coral calcium has been marketed as a wonder drug that can cure cancer, multiple sclerosis and a variety of other diseases. It's said to be better than regular calcium because the coral from which it is derived has trace amounts of other minerals. Many of the claims are based on the legendary long life and good health of Okinawans who supposedly drink water containing coral calcium.

However, two coral calcium marketers were ordered by the Federal Trade Commission to stop their infomercials and return money made as a result of misleading ads. Other companies still sell it; they just market coral calcium as a superior form of calcium, without describing it as a miracle cure-all.

I first learned about coral calcium from a relative who was taking it to prevent osteoporosis. Because of my gemological background, I knew that coral is just calcium carbonate, so I couldn't understand how coral calcium could be any better than calcium carbonate tablets. I decided to research it, and when I saw it at local pharmacies, health food stores and a vitamin shop, I examined the labels carefully.

Curiously, every brand of coral calcium I examined contained *supplemental* magnesium, usually in a ratio of two parts calcium to one part magnesium. This was the case even though the tablets were identified strictly as coral calcium. The magnesium was not part of the coral, it was added by the manufacturer in a laboratory. Usually vitamin D was also added. Plain calcium, however, was just labeled as calcium.

Is coral calcium better than other calcium? The answer depends on how you define "coral calcium." If you only mean the calcium carbonate in the tablet, the answer is no; it's not better than other calcium carbonate. However, if you're referring to the coral calcium tablet with the supplemental vitamin D and magnesium, the answer might be yes. Vitamin D is needed for optimal calcium absorption, and there is a significant amount of clinical evidence showing that calcium taken with vitamin D is more effective at decreasing bone loss than calcium taken alone, especially in areas where there is little winter sunshine. But you don't have to buy coral calcium to get a vitamin D supplement.

There isn't as much evidence about magnesium. Nevertheless, many health professionals have begun to recommend taking it with calcium when calcium supplements are warranted. Magnesium and vitamin D are also added to regular calcium tablets along with other nutrients, but the bottles are labeled as "calcium plus" or calcium plus magnesium and vitamin D, and so on. Magnesium and vitamin D are also sold separately. See next chapter for more information on magnesium, vitamin D and other nutrients.

You can learn more about the controversy regarding coral calcium at:
www.okinawaprogram.com/coral_calcium/coral-calcium.html
www.quackwatch.org/01QuackeryRelatedTopics/DSH/coral.html

Is Milk Bad for the Bones?

A surprising number of people have blamed dairy products for the high osteoporosis and fracture rates in the United States and other Westernized countries. They argue that countries with the lowest rates of milk consumption (e.g., Asian and African countries) have the lowest fracture rates; therefore it's better to avoid or restrict milk consumption.

Let's compare Asians to the average American:

◆ Asians typically eat more fruits and vegetables and a wider variety of them. These contain essential nutrients for bones.

◆ Asians are usually more active and spend more time walking and less time driving in cars.

◆ Asians typically eat a more balanced diet, including fish with bones, a good source of calcium, and soy products, a source of plant estrogens that is beneficial for bones.

◆ Asians eat less processed food.

◆ Asians are less dependent on bone-robbing drugs like corticosteroids.

◆ Many Asians live closer to the equator. The exposure to stronger UV rays from the sun helps their bodies produce more vitamin D, a nutrient that increases the absorption of calcium (see next chapter). Asians in northern latitudes often eat fish containing vitamin D.

◆ Seniors in Asia tend to have more household or farm-related responsibilities that require them to use their muscles. This in turn strengthens bone and improves balance. In America, it's more common to put seniors in assisted living centers where everything is done for them, and much of the time is spent sitting.

Is it any wonder that Asian countries have lower fracture rates than the United States?

Some people are concerned about an over-consumption of milk in America. Yet soda pop is more common than milk in the US. Fast food chains offer soft drinks with their "value meals," but seldom milk, unless specifically requested. Perhaps one reason osteoporosis seems to be rising in America is that children are drinking less and less milk and more and more non-nutritious drinks.

Dairy products are excellent sources of calcium, and numerous studies have shown them to be beneficial for bone health. Milk products are available in a variety of forms to fit your health needs and preferences: organic, fat-free, and low-fat. People with lactose intolerance might wish to try lactose-free milk such as Lactaid, calcium-fortified soy milk, or yogurt with active cultures in which the bacteria helps digest the lactose. Cheddar and Swiss cheese are also easier to digest than regular milk products.

Instead of devoting energy to criticizing milk, it would be more constructive to send a positive message like "Eat well-balanced meals with lots of fruits and vegetables."

9

Other Bone Nutrients

Even though calcium is a major component of bone, other minerals, vitamins, fatty acids and protein are also required for building and maintaining your skeletal structure. Some are listed below along with their bone-related functions:

Vitamin D   Promotes calcium absorption and bone mineralization; helps keep blood levels of calcium and phosphorus normal

Magnesium   Required for the absorption and metabolism of calcium; helps Vitamin D metabolism; stimulates the thyroid's production of the bone-building hormone, calcitonin; regulates the parathyroid gland, which controls the calcium in the blood

Vitamin K   Increases bone formation and decreases bone resorption, required for the production of osteocalcin (a bone protein)

Zinc   Required for the proper absorption of calcium and for bone formation; enhances the action of vitamin D

Boron   Improves the metabolism of both calcium and magnesium; can activate estrogen and vitamin D

Vitamin B_{12}   Helps the bone-building cells (osteoblasts) to function properly

If you have a well-rounded diet that includes food with the above nutrients, you will automatically get other nutrients that are also important for bone health. These include vitamins A, B_6, and C; folic acid, copper, phosphorous, fluoride, manganese, potassium, silica, and strontium. See Table 9.1 for U.S. recommended daily intakes of vitamins and elements.

The medical profession used to focus on calcium and vitamin D for the prevention of osteoporosis. That is changing. More and more articles are appearing in medical journals about the effects of other nutrients on bone density and fracture risk.

When some people read that a vitamin or mineral is beneficial for bone health, they are tempted to take it in large quantities. Curiously, this can have the opposite effect of weakening bones. A bone nutrient must be consumed in the proper amount together with other nutrients; these have a synergistic effect. The easiest and safest way of doing this is by eating

Table 9.1 Recommended intakes and limits for vitamins & food elements

Vitamins & elements	Recommended daily intakes for adults*	Tolerable Upper Intake Levels for adults*
A	700–900 mg (3000 IU)	3000 mg (10,000 IU)
B1 (thiamine)	1.1–1.2 mg	not determined
B2 (riboflavin)	1.1–1.3 mg	not determined
B3 (niacin)	14–16 mg	35 mg (debatable)
B6	1.3–1.7 mg	100 mg
B9 (folate, folic acid)	400 mcg	1000 mcg
B12 (cobalamin)	2.4 mcg	no adverse effects
C	75–90 mg	2000 mg
D	200–800 IU (5–15 mcg)	2000 IU (50 mcg)
E	11–15 mg (16.5–22.5 IU)	1000 mg (1500 IU)
K	90 micrograms	not determined
boron	not established	20 mg
calcium	1000–1200 mg	2500 mg
chromium	20–30 mcg	not determined
copper	900 mcg	10,000 mcg
fluoride	3–4 mg	10 mg
iodine	150 mcg	1100 mcg
iron	8–18 mg	45 mg
magnesium	320–420 mcg	depends on the source
manganese	1.8–2.3 mg	11 mg
phosphorous	700 mg	3000–4000 mg
potassium	4700 mg	not determined
selenium	55 mg	400 mcg
zinc	8–11 mg	40 mg

Source: Food & Nutrient Board, Institute of Medicine, US National Academies

* Pregnant and lactating women usually have higher requirements

IU = international units, mg = milligrams, mcg = micrograms (same as μg) nutritious food. Supplements are helpful when medical conditions and dietary restrictions prevent you from getting the required nutrients from food. The rest of this chapter discusses in more detail the benefits, sources and side effects of some of the most important bone nutrients. You'll understand it better if you know the following terms and abbreviations, which were developed by the US Food and Drug Administration (FDA) and the Institute of Medicine of the National Academy of Sciences:

Recommended Dietary Allowance (RDA): the average daily intake that is sufficient to meet the nutrient requirements of nearly all (97-98%) healthy individuals in each age and gender group

Adequate Intake (AI):amount needed to maintain a nutritional state of adequacy in nearly all members of a specific age and gender group. An AI is established when there is insufficient scientific data available to establish a RDA for specific age/gender groups

Estimated Average Requirement (EAR): the intake value estimated to meet the nutritional needs in 50% of an age and gender-specific group

Tolerable Upper Intake Levels (UL): the maximum daily intake unlikely to result in adverse effects

Dietary Reference Intake (DRI): A generic term used to refer to at least three reference values: EAR, RDA and UL. It's a new approach to determining nutrient reference values. The Food and Nutrition Board of the National Academies of Sciences has worked with Health Canada to set the new recommended intake values.

Daily Value (DV): reference numbers developed by the Food and Drug Administration (FDA) to help consumers determine if a food contains a lot or a little of a specific nutrient. A food that supplies 20% or more of that nutrient is high in that nutrient.

Microgram (mcg or μg): one millionth of a gram; "mcg" is the preferred abbreviation because "μg" can be confused with "mg" when handwritten.

Milligram (mg): One thousandth of a gram

International Unit (IU): an internationally accepted amount of a substance such as a vitamin or hormone, which produces a specified effect when tested. The quantity varies depending on the substance. For example, 1 IU of Vitamin D = .025 mcg, but 1 IU of Vitamin A = .3 mcg.

(The above definitions and much of the material in this chapter is from the websites of the Office of Dietary Supplements of the US National Institutes of Health, **www.ods.od.nih.gov,** the US Department of Agriculture, **www.nal.usda.gov/fnic/foodcomp/Data/** and the Food and Nutrition Board, Institute of Medicine Project, National Academies at **www.iom.edu/subpage.asp?id=13063**

Vitamin D

The major function of vitamin D is to maintain normal blood levels of calcium and phosphorous. It is a fat-soluble vitamin, which means it requires some dietary fat for absorption, but much of it is made by the body upon exposure to the ultraviolet rays of the sun.

Vitamin D can help reduce hip fractures. Without it, bones become thin, brittle or misshapen, and children can develop a disease known as rickets. A vitamin D deficiency can be caused by pollution and the heavy use of sunscreens because they block UV rays from the sun that trigger vitamin D synthesis in the skin. People from cultures that always wear robes and head garments or who live in northern latitudes, where there is little winter sunshine, are also susceptible to vitamin D deficiency.

According to the Office of Dietary Supplements of the National Institutes of Health, "Ten to fifteen minutes of sun exposure at least two times per week to the face, arms, hands, or back without sunscreen is usually sufficient to provide adequate vitamin D." After 15 minutes of unblocked sunlight, you can protect your skin from the negative consequences of excessive sun exposure by applying a sunscreen of a sun protection factor (SPF) of at least 15. For more information see:

www.ods.od.nih.gov/factsheets/vitamind.asp#h2

Some people wonder if you can use sun lamps as a substitute for sunshine. In her book *Strong Women, Strong Bones* (p 285). Miriam Nelson PhD says that a tanning lamp can be used as a source of vitamin D because the special light bulb triggers the same reaction in your skin as the sun. However, she cautions that tanning lamps, like over-exposure to the sun, carry a risk of skin cancer. Therefore a vitamin D supplement might be a better choice.

Major sources of vitamin D: sunshine (primary source), cold saltwater fish like salmon, tuna, shrimp and halibut, cod liver oil, fortified cereal, fortified milk and many calcium supplements

Recommended Adequate Intake of vitamin D (increases as we get older)

200 IU or 5 micrograms — birth to age 50 (IU=International Units)

400 IU or 10 micrograms — ages 51 to 70)

600 IU or 15 micrograms — ages 71 and older

Tolerable Upper Intake Level of vitamin D per day:

1000 IU or 25 micrograms — 0 to 12 months,

2000 IU or 50 micrograms — ages above a year

Symptoms of vitamin D toxicity: nausea, vomiting, poor appetite, constipation, weakness and high blood levels of calcium, which in turn cause confusion and heart rhythm abnormalities. Calcinosis, the deposition of too much calcium in the soft tissues such as the kidney, can also be caused by vitamin D toxicity resulting from excessive cod liver oil or supplements.

Vitamin D content in major food sources

Food	IU	Food	IU
cod liver oil 1 tbsp, 15 ml	1,360	salmon 3½ oz, 99gms	360
mackerel 3½ oz, 99g	345	canned sardines 1¾ oz, 49 g	250
tuna in oil 3 oz, 85 g	200	fortified milk 1 cup, 237 ml	98
fortified margarine 1 tbsp	60	1 egg, vitamin D is in yolk	20
liver, beef 3 ½ oz, 99g	15	Swiss cheese 1oz, 28 g	12

Source: Office of Dietary Supplements, US National Institutes of Health
www.ods.od.nih.gov/factsheets/vitamind.asp

Magnesium

Magnesium is the fourth most abundant mineral in the body after calcium, phosphorous and potassium; and 50 percent of it is found in the bones. Besides making the bones stronger, it also regulates your heartbeat and blood sugar, promotes normal blood pressure, supports the immune system, and helps maintain normal nerve and muscle function. It even helps alleviate arthritis.

Calcium and magnesium work together; for example, if you have a deficiency of either mineral, you might have an irregular heartbeat because calcium is instrumental in causing muscles like the heart to contract, whereas magnesium allows them to relax. Likewise, a deficiency of either calcium or magnesium can prevent proper absorption of the other element. You must have an adequate intake of each of these two elements for your body to function properly.

Even though published works by nutritionists (e.g. Nan Fuchs, PhD; Susan Brown, PhD) often recommend taking magnesium in conjunction with calcium, few books or articles by medical doctors advise magnesium supplementation. However, that is changing. For example, in his book

"Beautiful Bones Without Hormones (p 88)," orthopedist Leon Root says, "In many cases where calcium intake is sufficient, magnesium supplements may be even more important than calcium supplements." According to Dr. Root, the appropriate calcium to magnesium ratio is 2:1, especially if you already have osteoporosis. If you have arthritis or a heart condition, however, you may need more magnesium. He advises that you ask your doctor what the appropriate calcium/magnesium ratio is for you.

The website of the Office of Dietary Supplements says, "Some evidence suggests that magnesium deficiency may be an additional risk factor for postmenopausal osteoporosis. . . . Several human studies have suggested that magnesium supplementation may improve bone mineral density." (www.ods.od.nih.gov/factsheets/magnesium.asp)

Do not take magnesium with tetracycline antibiotics. The magnesium decreases the absorption of tetracycline. Check with your pharmacist and doctor before taking over-the-counter drugs and nutritional supplements, especially if you take medications or have medical problems.

Major sources of magnesium: dark green vegetables, whole-grains, legumes, nuts, chocolate, magnesium containing-laxatives and antacids

Recommended Dietary Allowances (RDA) of magnesium:

    80 mg — 1 to 3 years of age
130 mg — 4 to 8 years
240 mg — 9 to 13 years
310 to 420 — 14+

Tolerable Upper Intake Levels (UL) for magnesium: There's no UL for dietary intake of magnesium. It's safe to get any amount of magnesium from food. The Office of Dietary Supplements states that the UL for *supplemental* magnesium is 350 mg for people aged 9 and above. Some nutritionists probably consider this UL too low. In *Better Bones, Better Body* (pp 88), nutritionist Susan Brown, PhD says that recent large-scale balance studies indicate that we might actually need about 450 mg of magnesium a day.

Side effects of excess magnesium: diarrhea, nausea, appetite loss, muscle weakness, extremely low blood pressure, and irregular heartbeat. If an excess occurs, it's generally caused by taking too many magnesium containing laxatives or antacids. Magnesium *in food* is safe even in large quantities.

Symptoms and effects of magnesium deficiency: Early signs are nausea, vomiting, fatigue and weakness. Later it can lead to numbness, tingling, muscle cramps, seizures, abnormal heart rhythms, coronary spasms, aortic calcification and low blood calcium and potassium. Kidney stones can also develop as a result of inadequate magnesium, especially if you have a high intake of calcium.

Some causes of magnesium deficiency other than diet: alcoholism, diuretics, certain antibiotics, poorly controlled diabetes, Chrohn's disease and other chronic malabsorptive problems

Magnesium content in some major food sources

Food	mg	Food	mg
halibut 3 oz, 85 g	90	almonds 1 oz, 28 g	80
cashews 1 oz, 28 g	75	soybeans ½ cup, 113 g	75
spinach ½ cup, 119 ml	75	shredded wheat 2 biscuits	55
baked potato with skin	50	peanuts 1 oz, 28 g	50
yogurt 1 cup, 237 ml	45	brown rice ½ cup, 113 g	40
avocado ½ cup, 119 ml	35	lentils ½ cup, 113 g	35
beans ½ cup, 119 ml	35	one banana	30
chocolate milk 1cup, 237 ml	35	milk chocolate 1.5 oz, 42g	28
fat-free milk 1cup, 237 ml	27	whole milk 1cup, 237 ml	24

Source: Office of Dietary Supplements, US National Institutes of Health
www.ods.od.nih.gov/factsheets/magnesium.asp

Vitamin K

Vitamin K is a fat-soluble vitamin that is best known for its role in helping blood to clot (the letter K comes from the Danish word "koagulation"). However, recent studies have found another benefit— women with higher vitamin K intakes have higher bone densities and lower fracture rates. According to an article on vitamin K in the October 2004 issue of *American Journal of Clinical Nutrition* (p 1075), the exact role of vitamin K is unclear, but it has been shown to increase the production of cells that build new bone (osteoblasts).

Major sources of vitamin K: Dark green leafy vegetables are the best sources of vitamin K. One-half cup of boiled kale, turnip greens, collards or spinach has over five times the Daily Value (DV) of vitamin K. It's also found in vegetable oils such as olive, canola and soybean oil.

Adequate Intake Level (AI) of vitamin K: 90–120 micrograms (mcg). The Daily Value (D.V.) is 65–80 micrograms per day for adults.

Vitamin K toxicity and interactions: Vitamin K is relatively safe for people who do not need blood thinners. The National Academies state that no upper limit has been established. According to the Merck Manual, vitamin K_1 (Phylloquinone) is not toxic at 500 times the RDA. However a vitamin K precursor called menadione can cause anemia in excessive amounts.

People taking blood thinners such as Coumadin® (warfarin) should keep their intake of vitamin K as consistent as possible because sudden increases in vitamin K from foods such as dark green leafy vegetables may decrease the effect of the drug. In addition, some antibiotics can either lower vitamin K levels or interfere with the action of Coumadin®. Patients taking the drug should consult with their physician before using any dietary supplement, including vitamin K.

More detailed information for people taking Coumadin® and vitamin K can be found at www.ods.od.nih.gov/factsheets/cc/coumadin1.pdf of the National Institutes of Health.

Vitamin K content in major food sources, % Daily Value (DV)

Food	% DV	Food	% DV
kale, boiled ½ cup	660	spinach, boiled ½ cup	560
turnip greens ½ cup	530	collards, boiled ½ cup	520
Swiss chard ½ cup	360	brussels sprouts ½ cup	190
raw spinach 1 cup	180	raw turnip greens 1 cup	170
green leaf lettuce 1 cup	125	chopped raw broccoli 1 cup	110
endive lettuce 1 cup	70	romaine lettuce 1 cup	70

Source: Office of Dietary Supplements, US National Institutes of Health

Boron

Boron is a nonmetallic element that occurs naturally only as a compound such as borax or boric acid. Boron compounds are used to produce glass, fire retardants, cosmetics, photographic materials, laundry products and some pesticides.

Only since 1987 have scientists found boron to be important for bone health and the prevention of osteoporosis. The body needs boron to metabolize and use bone-building agents such as calcium, magnesium, vitamin D and estrogen.

Major sources of boron: fruits, vegetables, nuts, beans and some tap water. It's measured in milligrams.

Recommended Dietary Allowance of boron:. No RDA, AI or EAR has been established by the US government for boron, but recent research suggests that 2 to 3 mg per day is probably the optimum intake (p 120 of *Beautiful Bones Without Hormones* by orthopedist Leon Root).

Tolerable Upper Intake Level of boron per day:

11 mg — 9 to 13 years

17 mg — 14 to 18 years

20 mg — 19 + years

Boron that occurs naturally in food is safe. No adverse effects from boron have been reported in areas where as much as 40 mg of boron are consumed daily in food. It's when excess boron is consumed from additives or supplementation that health problems can occur.

Symptoms of boron toxicity: Gastrointestinal problems, nasal congestion, skin redness and loss of body hair. According to the U.S. Agency for Toxic Substances and Disease Registry (www.atsdr.cdc.gov), ingesting large amounts of boron over short periods of time can harm the stomach, intestines, liver, and brain. As a result, boron has been outlawed for use as a food preservative.

Foods containing boron: Foods high in boron include: almonds, apricots, avocados, dates, hazel nuts, kidney beans, peanut butter, raisins and wine. The best way to get adequate boron is to eat several servings of fruits, vegetables and nuts per day.

Zinc

Besides playing a central role in bone formation, the mineral zinc supports the immune system, helps maintain your sense of taste and smell, promotes normal growth, and stimulates the activity of about 100 enzymes. It's also needed for DNA synthesis and wound healing. Low levels of zinc are associated with osteoporosis and stunted growth.

Major sources of zinc: Oysters, red meat and poultry have the highest amount of zinc per serving, but beans, nuts, whole grains, fortified breakfast cereals and dairy products are also good sources of zinc.

Recommended Dietary Allowance of zinc: 8–12 mg per day for adults and children ages 9 and above. Pregnant and breast-feeding women need more than the average person.

Tolerable Upper Intake Level (UL) of zinc: 40 mg per day for ages 19+

Symptoms and consequences of zinc toxicity (have occurred with intakes of over 150 mg per day): reduced immune function, reduced levels of good cholesterol (HDL), reduced absorption of copper, altered iron function. **People with kidney disease should not take zinc supplements.** They should get zinc from dietary sources.

Zinc content in major food sources

Food	mg	Food	mg
oysters 6 medium	16	lean beef shank 3 oz, 85 g	8.9
lean beef chuck roast 85 g	7.4	lean beef tenderloin 85 g	7.4
lean pork shoulder 3 oz, 85 g	4.2	fortified breakfast cereal with 25% daily value ¾ c	3.8
meat of one chicken leg	2.7	lean pork loin roast 85 g	2.2
plain non-fat yogurt 1 cup	2.2	baked beans ½ cup, 113 g	1.8
cashews 1 oz, 28g	1.6	low-fat fruit yogurt 1 cup	1.6
pecans 1 oz, 28 g	1.4	almonds, walnuts 1 oz, 28g	1.0
milk 1 cup, 237 ml	0.9	½ chicken breast, skinless	0.9

Source: Office of Dietary Supplements, US National Institutes of Health

Vitamin B$_{12}$

Vitamin B$_{12}$ is best known for stimulating the formation of red blood cells in the bone marrow. This water-soluble vitamin also helps maintain a healthy nervous system and stimulates bone-building cells (osteoblasts). Thanks to some recent research, this water-soluble vitamin is becoming better known for its role in improving bone quality.

One double-blind, randomized study of a group of 628 Japanese stroke victims 65 years or older found that giving stroke patients vitamins B$_{12}$ and folic acid decreased their risk of hip fracture. *Journal of the American Medical Association.* March 2, 2005, Vol. 293, No. 9, pp. 1082–1087.

Another study of 2576 people found that both men and women with low levels of B$_{12}$ had average lower bone densities than people with higher levels of B$_{12}$. That study was conducted by the USDA Human Nutrition Research Center at Tufts University. *Journal of Bone and Mineral Research*, 2005 Jan;20(1):152-8.

Vitamin B$_{12}$ works very closely with vitamin B$_6$ and folic acid (a compound of the B complex group, which is also called folate and vitamin B$_9$). All three play a role in bone health. If folic acid is taken alone, for example, it can decrease the absorption of vitamin B$_{12}$. Consequently, it's advisable to take these B-complex vitamins in combination with each other. The Office of Dietary Supplements states "Folic acid intake from food and supplements should not exceed 1,000 micrograms per day in healthy individuals because large amounts of folic acid can trigger the damaging effects of vitamin B$_{12}$ deficiency. Adults older than 50 years who take a folic acid supplement should ask their physician or qualified health care provider about their need for vitamin B$_{12}$ supplementation."

Major sources of vitamin B$_{12}$: animal foods including shellfish, meat, fish, poultry, eggs, milk, and milk products. Fortified breakfast cereals are a good source of vitamin B$_{12}$ for vegetarians.

Recommended Dietary Allowance (RDA) of B$_{12}$: 2.4– 2.8 micrograms (mcg) for adults. The Daily Value (DV) is 6.0 micrograms.

Tolerable Upper Intake Level of B$_{12}$: None has been established by the Institute of Medicine of the National Academy of Sciences for vitamin B$_{12}$ because it has a very low potential for toxicity. The Institute states that "no adverse effects have been associated with excess vitamin B$_{12}$ intake from food and supplements in healthy individuals" In fact, the Institute recommends that adults over 50 years of age get most of their vitamin B$_{12}$ from vitamin supplements or fortified food because of the high incidence of impaired absorption of B_{12} from animal foods in this age group. (From http://ods.od.nih.gov/factsheets/vitaminb12.asp#h11)

Even though vitamin B_{12} is relatively safe in high doses, this is not true of some of the other B complex vitamins. For example, too much vitamin B_6 from supplements can result in nerve damage to the arms and legs. The upper tolerable intake level of vitamin B_6 is 100 mg per day.

If folic acid is taken alone, it can decrease the absorption of vitamin B_{12}. The Office of Dietary Supplements states "Folic acid intake from food and supplements should not exceed 1,000 micrograms daily in healthy individuals because large amounts of folic acid can trigger the damaging effects of vitamin B_{12} deficiency. Adults older than 50 years who take a folic acid supplement should ask their physician or qualified health care provider about their need for vitamin B_{12} supplementation."

Signs and symptoms of vitamin B_{12} deficiency: Anemia, dementia, fatigue, loss of appetite, fatigue, weight loss, confusion, poor memory, depression, numbness, problems maintaining balance, tingling in the hands and feet (Many of these symptoms can also result from other medical conditions). B_{12} deficiency in infants can result in permanent neurologic damage. Therefore the Office of Dietary Supplements of the National Institutes of Health advises: **"Mothers who follow a strict vegetarian diet should consult with a pediatrician regarding appropriate vitamin B_{12} supplementation for their infants and children."**

Vitamin B_{12} content in major food sources

Food	mcg	Food	mcg
mollusks, clams 3 oz, 85 g	84	beef liver 1 slice	47.9
100% fortified cereal	6.0	wild rainbow trout 85 g	5.4
farmed rainbow trout 85 g	4.2	sockeye salmon 85 g	4.2
top sirloin beef 3 oz, 85 g	2.4	beef taco	1.6
double patty cheeseburger	1.9	plain skim yogurt 1 cup	1.4
tuna 3 oz, 85 g	1.0	milk 1cup, 0.24 liter	0.9
roasted ham 3 oz, 85 g	0.6	1 egg	0.6
pasteurized cheese slice	0.3	½ chicken breast meat	0.3

Source: Office of Dietary Supplements of the US National Institutes of Health

Plant-derived Estrogens

Soybeans, chickpeas, lentils and other legumes contain substances called **phytoestrogens**, which mimic the hormone estrogen, but appear to have no harmful side effects ("phyto" means plant). Japanese women, who consume a lot of soy products, have much lower incidences of osteoporosis, breast cancer, heart disease and hot flashes than women in the United States. The blood levels of phytoestrogens in the Japanese are also much higher. The plant-derived estrogens in soybeans are a class of phyto-estrogens called **isoflavones**.

Harris McIlwain, MD, chairman of the Florida Osteoporosis board, says "while studies are few, findings support that eating soy foods strengthens bone." In his book, *Reversing Osteopenia* (p.69), he mentions a study on Chinese women published in the October 2003 issue of *Osteoporosis International*, which concluded that "soybean and isoflavone ingestion results in a modest but significant increase in hip bone mineral density and higher overall body bone mineral density."

Felicia Cosman, MD, clinical director of the National Osteoporosis Foundation, says that studies in monkeys have shown that phytoestrogens from soy products called isoflavones inhibit bone loss and decrease atherosclerosis. However, Cosman warns that the effects of high doses of isoflavones obtained in pill form may differ from those of the lower doses consumed in the diet, and their safety particularly for the breast and uterus has not been determined. Therefore, Cosman concludes that while it may be reasonable to recommend using moderate amounts of soy products in the diet, "it is not recommended that people consume isoflavone-derivative pills, particularly for a prolonged period of time" (*What Your Doctor May Not Tell You about Osteoporosis*, pp 93, 94).

Cosman also advises against the use of **ipriflavone**, a synthetic derivative of isoflavones, available over the counter without a doctor's prescription as a supplement for preventing osteoporosis. She says that a study performed on more that four hundred women with osteoporosis indicated that ipriflavone does not improve bone density or bone turnover; nor does it reduce the occurrence of vertebral fractures. Moreover, in a significant number of women, it actually produced a reduction in the number of lymphocytes (a type of white blood cell that fights infection). Consequently, ipriflavone may be dangerous.

In sum, eat soy products, and get phytoestrogens from food instead of relying on pills. Plant estrogens are also found in lentils, chick peas and some other legumes but the amounts are negligible. When cooked the phytoestrogen content decreases. See table below:

Isoflavone content of selected foods in mg/100 grams of edible portion

soy milk, skin or film (Foo jook or yuba), raw	193.88
soy flour, full-fat raw	177
soybeans, raw, content varies depending on source country	87–150
soybeans, mature, dry roasted	128.35
tempeh (a fermented tofu-like food made from cooked soybeans)	62.50
miso soup, dry mix	60.39
soybeans, mature, boiled without salt	54.66
soybean chips	54.16
soy milk, skin or film (Foo jook or yuba), cooked	50.70
miso	42.55
soybean curd cheese	28.20
tofu, content varies depending on type and brand	22–33
tofu yogurt	16.30
soy hot dog (frozen, unprepared)	15.00
bacon, meatless	12.10
soy milk fluid	9.65
soy noodles, flat	8.50
Green Giant Harvest Burger, all vegetable protein patties	8.22
soy cheese, mozzarella	7.70
split peas, raw, mature,	2.42
USDA beef patties with VVP, frozen, cooked	1.86
peanuts, raw	0.26
chickpeas (garbanzo beans) raw	0.10

green tea and Twinings jasmine tea	0.05
kidney beans, raw mature	0.03
lentils, raw mature	0.01
kidney beans, cooked mature	0.00

Source: USDA-Iowa State Database on the Isoflavone Content of Foods – 1999
www.nal.usda.gov/fnic/foodcomp/Data/isoflav/isfl_tbl.pdf

Nutrients that can Be Both Good and Bad for Bones

Nutrients that help build and strengthen bone can sometimes make them more susceptible to breakage or osteoporosis when taken to excess. Three of these nutrients include:

Excess vitamin A: This oil-soluble vitamin is essential for normal bone development and proper metabolism of calcium. But if you take too much vitamin A (also called retinol), it can cause reduced bone mineral density, birth defects, and liver abnormalities. Even though vitamin A toxicity can occur from regularly consuming large amounts of liver, most cases of it result from an excess of vitamin A supplementation.

A nurses' health study and two Swedish studies have found an association between excess intake of vitamin A and increased fracture risk. Researchers suspect that excess vitamin A may impair the ability of vitamin D to promote calcium absorption. You can get more detailed information at www.ods.od.nih.gov/factsheets/vitamina.asp#h6. After reaching this website of the Office of Dietary Supplements of the National Institute of Health, scroll down to the section entitled "Vitamin A and osteoporosis."

According to the National Institute of Health, the Tolerable Upper Intake level of vitamin A for adults is 3000 mcg or 10,000 IU. The Recommended Dietary Allowance (RDA) for adults ranges from 700–1300 mcg or 2330–4335 IU per day. The safest form of vitamin A supplementation is beta carotene, a substance that the body converts to vitamin A. The best way to get adequate vitamin A is from food such as liver or darkly colored fruits and vegetables. Carrots, sweet potatoes, spinach, cantaloupe and mangos are especially high in vitamin A. One carrot can give you more than four times the RDA of vitamin A.

Excess protein: Calcium is required for protein metabolism. Therefore if protein intake is high and calcium intake is low, calcium is drawn out of the bones, and a loss of the mineral and bone can result. This is evidenced by the fact that as the consumption of protein increases; the urinary excretion of calcium also increases.

The recommended dietary allowance (RDA) for protein is from 46–56 grams (1.62–1.98 oz) per day. Nutritionist Susan Brown, PhD says that people consuming 45 grams of protein and 500 mg of calcium have been found to be in positive calcium balance, which means that their protein intake did not cause a loss of calcium from the body (p. 124 of *Better Bones, Better Body*). A higher consumption of protein requires a higher consumption of calcium.

Nevertheless, protein is important for bone health. Bone is a composite material consisting of mineral crystals bound to protein. The protein provides strength and resilience so that the skeleton can absorb impact without breaking. A structure made only of mineral would be more brittle and break more easily, whereas a structure made only of protein would be soft and bend too easily (p.18 of *Bone Health and Osteoporosis: A Report of the Surgeon General*).

Inadequate protein intakes have been associated with poor recovery from osteoporotic fractures, and serum albumin values (an indicator of protein nutritional status) have been found to be inversely related to hip fracture risk. A proper balance of bone nutrients is important for the prevention of osteoporosis. Sources: Linus Pauling Institute.
http://lpi.oregonstate.edu/infocenter/minerals/calcium/index.html
(scroll down to "Protein")
www.susanbrownphd.com/hot_topics/protein_bone_health.htm
"Protein and Bone Health a Paradox Unraveled"

Excess fluoride: Fluoride makes bones and teeth harder and denser. However, an excessive amount of it can lead to an increased risk of hip and peripheral stress fractures, abnormal bone growth and mottling of the teeth. Consequently, fluoride supplementation is seldom recommended for osteoporosis prevention. You can safely get adequate amounts of fluoride from food and beverages such as fish, eggs, tea, milk, lettuce, cabbage, oats, whole wheat and some public water. For more information on fluoride see *What Your Doctor May Not Tell you About Osteoporosis* by Felicia Cosman, MD (pp 228, 229) and *Osteoporosis Handbook* by Sydney Lou Bonnick, MD (pp 188, 189).

In essence, too much of a good thing can be harmful. Avoid flooding your body with too many supplements, eat a well-balanced diet with *moderate* amounts of protein, and try to get bone nutrients primarily from food.

10

Fighting Osteoporosis and Losing Weight

I was seated at a banquet next to a youthful-looking blond (let's call her Sue) and we were discussing our work. When I told her my next book would be on osteoporosis, Sue said that her bones were "a crumblin," so she was taking Fosamax. Her doctor had suggested a bone density test earlier than usual because she had been a model and was thin-boned with a family history of osteoporosis. The test confirmed that she had a bad case of osteoporosis.

Many ex-models who have been on severe diets end up with osteoporosis as a result of poor nutrition during their formative years. Besides taking Fosamax, Sue now exercises regularly and eats a well-balanced diet. Nevertheless, it's hard to build bone after you've reached peak bone mass in your thirties. That's why osteoporosis prevention must start early.

Osteoporosis, Body Weight **and** Dieting

One advantage of being overweight is that you may be at lower risk of osteoporosis and bone fracture. Extra weight can put an extra load on the bones, thus stimulating bone formation as weight training and exercise do. The extra fat may also act as protective padding if you fall. Unfortunately, excessive weight creates other health problems such as heart disease, osteoarthritis and diabetes.

Extra body weight can have a detrimental effect on your bones if it leads to excessive dieting, yoyo dieting or unhealthy fad diets.

In her book *Strong Women Strong Bones* (p 54), Miriam Nelson, PhD, states that frequent cycles of losing and regaining 15 or more pounds increases your risk of osteoporosis. Rapid weight loss is especially detrimental to bone because it prompts the release of parathyroid hormone, which increases bone-dissolving activity in your body.

Nelson says the best ways to counter these effects is to lose weight slowly (no more that a pound or two per week) and to do aerobic exercise and strength training.

High protein diets can also lead to bone loss. In *The Osteoporosis Handbook* (pp 18–19), Dr. Sydney Bonnick says that excessive protein in the diet can increase calcium loss in the urine. Whenever you double the amount of protein you eat, the calcium loss in your urine increases by 50%. Calcium supplements can help counter the loss.

Bonnick also states that studies have clearly linked high dietary protein intake to the risk of hip fractures. Nevertheless, protein is essential for building bone and muscle; too little protein has also been linked to bone fractures. The key is to eat a balanced diet without excessive protein.

Osteoporosis and Eating Disorders

Anorexia nervosa, a type of self-starvation, is the most serious eating disorder. It's most commonly found in adolescent girls and young women, many of whom are athletic and overly concerned about their weight. They have an unrealistic perception of their body size and an abnormal fear of being fat. Anorexia leads to osteoporosis through inadequate nutrient intake and severe weight loss. This in turn results in decreased estrogen and irregular or absent menstrual cycles, a condition called **amenorrhea**. If left untreated, anorexia can lead to death. It's important to find the underlying psychological cause of the disorder.

Bulimia is an eating disorder that involves repeatedly gorging oneself with food and then purging it with laxatives or by vomiting. The body becomes depleted of water, potassium and other minerals including calcium, which is needed for proper bone growth. Bulimics, however, may be of normal weight and may continue menstruating. Consequently they are not as likely to get osteoporosis as anorexic women.

In *Strong Women Strong Bones (pp 54–58),* Miriam Nelson, PhD says that up to 30 percent of female college varsity athletes have some form of eating disorder. She and her Tufts University colleagues recruited twenty-eight women runners in their twenties and thirties that ran at least 25 miles a week. However, eleven had not menstruated for at least a year and had a significantly lower bone density than the menstruating women. Further research showed that the eleven non-menstruating women had disordered patterns of eating—for example, some had only one meal a day or consumed many foods in exceptionally tiny portions.

Some reports of low bone mass and irregular periods in women athletes may lead people to incorrectly conclude that engaging in a lot of exercise is harmful. Inadequate nutrition appears to be the source of the problems, not exercise. Male athletes, who are usually hearty eaters, have stronger bones and muscles than their non athletic counterparts.

How I Lost Weight Fighting Osteoporosis

While doing research on osteoporosis, I read in some sources that diets with a high acid-forming effect can deplete calcium reserves in the body and cause bone-thinning (e.g., pp 294–303 of *Better Bones, Better Body* by nutritionist Susan Brown). Fruits and vegetables, for instance, are supposed to have an alkaline-forming effect on the body chemistry, while refined sugar and protein have an acid-forming effect.

I also read that you can determine the acidity of your body by testing your saliva or urine with pH hydrion paper strips when you first wake up.

To reduce my body's acidity, I decreased my protein and gave up all products with sugar. I tried to measure my progress using PH testing strips, but the results were inconclusive.

However, the experiment had an unexpected effect. I lost five pounds in one month. I didn't want to lose the weight, though, because I'm already sufficiently thin. Consequently, I resumed my previous eating habits.

How You Can Lose Weight, Yet Get Adequate Nutrition

A few months after trying to eliminate sugar from my diet, a friend told me she had lost weight by eliminating foods with white flour and refined sugar from her diet. Otherwise she ate mostly what she wanted within a certain caloric range (1200 calories). She also attended a support group of others who followed the same diet. Those who stuck to the diet lost weight and kept it off.

Here are some other things you can do to lose weight, yet get adequate nutrition.

◆ **Eat a heart-healthy diet very low in saturated and trans fat.** For example, eat lean meat, use fat-free or at least low-fat dairy products, and avoid junk food like chips, candy bars and cookies.

◆ **Eat a higher percentage of fruits and vegetables and other fiber-rich foods like beans and whole grains.** These foods have bone-building nutrients, and the fiber can help you feel full with fewer calories. Fiber also helps food move more quickly through your body.

◆ **Be active and increase the duration of your exercise.** Body activity not only burns calories. It can also raise your metabolism rate. I suspect the reason that I can eat a high-calorie diet without gaining weight is because I'm active and exercise a lot.

A Wish List for Eating Out

It would be nice if people could eat out and get calcium-rich dairy foods without a lot of fat. But it's hard to do. Restaurants offer few options for people who want to reduce their intake of fat. Below are some items that would be nice to find at restaurants and food outlets.

◆ Baked potatoes with fat-free sour cream. (Good brands of fat-free sour cream can be just as tasty and creamy as the regular varieties).

◆ Low-fat and/or fat-free ice-cream. If they are available at ice cream shops, there is typically only one flavor, usually vanilla.

◆ Mexican food with low-fat cheese and fat-free sour cream

◆ Fat-free or 1% milk-fat milk

◆ Fat-free or low-fat cottage cheese

◆ Tuna and chicken salads and sandwiches made with fat-free sour cream or yogurt instead of mayonnaise. They taste just as good.

◆ Pizza with low-fat cheese

Considering the number of people who want to lose weight and/or prevent heart disease, it's surprising that dairy products with cream or whole milk are usually the only ones served in restaurants. Hopefully, one day that will change.

11

Osteoporosis Drugs: Pros & Cons

I don't like taking drugs. During the last twenty years, I've only taken two prescription drugs—an antibiotic, which I took for just one week, and the osteoporosis drug Fosamax® (alendronate), which I started taking in the summer of 2003. I don't even take aspirin, Tylenol, or herbal supplements.

The only reason I considered taking alendronate is because I hadn't been able to maintain my bone mass with natural methods such as diet, exercise and calcium. Nevertheless, I wouldn't have taken alendronate, had I not first done research and talked to people about it. Osteoporosis medications are optional drugs. You can live without them. Before taking such drugs, you should research them. The next section lists reasons why I followed my doctor's advice to take alendronate.

Taking Alendronate (Fosamax), a Personal Decision

I first learned about alendronate after my mother had a bone density test. It was one of the drugs suggested by her doctor, but she never took it. The following combination of events and factors led me to take it instead.

◆ Several years ago, a former neighbor broke her hip and arm after losing her balance while picking up a bottle. Her orthopedist said she had osteoporosis and recommended alendronate, which she still takes. She's never had any side effects and she credits alendronate for preventing her from having any more fractures. Even though she's fallen several times because of poor eyesight, she's only suffered bruises.

Witnessing her customer testimonial firsthand made a greater impression on me than any doctor recommendation could.

◆ Ever since my neighbor started taking alendronate, I've read whatever I've seen about it. With the exception of literature from marketers of bone-boosting products, most has been favorable.

For example, Felicia Cosman, MD, clinical director of the National Osteoporosis Foundation, states that alendronate "increases bone mass throughout the skeleton more than any other antiresorptive medicine and reduces bone turnover more potently than any other medicine" (page 203 of *What Your Doctor May Not Tell You about Osteoporosis).*

She goes on to say that all of the results concerning alendronate come from well-designed randomized controlled trials. The largest study, the Fracture Intervention Trial (FIT), enrolled over 2000 women. The results indicated that alendronate reduced the risk of hip, spine and wrist fractures. However, medical professionals disagree about the significance of the decreased fracture rates.

Cosman has seen clinical evidence that backs up the findings of the trials. For example, one of her patients came to her clinic with severe back pain due to multiple vertebral fractures that had occurred during the preceding year. After she had been on alendronate for about six months, the pain began to cease, and she hasn't had any fractures since.

◆ A relative, who was on alendronate, got her bone density results about the same time as I did. Her bone density in the spine and hip had increased over the same time period that mine had gone down. This was in spite of the fact that I exercised more, had a healthier diet and got more calcium and vitamin D. She did not have any side effects from alendronate.

◆ My dentist told me my gums were receding a little as a result of some bone loss in my jaw, which is visible in my dental x-rays. I figured that alendronate might be the most effective way of preventing additional bone loss since weight training does not normally target the jawbone.

Keeping ones natural teeth is also important. After people get dentures, they lose bone in their jaw, probably because they're not able to chew with as much force. My dentist says that people with dentures only have 20 to 25 percent of the biting pressure of people with natural teeth and healthy gums.

◆ The physician's prescribing leaflet that was included in the sample my doctor gave me had convincing evidence that alendronate was effective.

◆ I felt more comfortable with a drug that has been on the market over ten years than with the newer osteoporosis medications, which have been used by fewer people for a shorter amount of time. However, if I'd had a bad reaction to alendronate, I would have tried a newer medication.

Why Take Bone Drugs Before You Have Osteoporosis?

Opinions differ among medical professionals as to when is the best time to start drug therapy for the prevention and treatment of osteoporosis. However, most would agree that both pregnant and nursing women and women who plan to have children should not take alendronate and the similar drugs risedronate (Actonel®) and ibandronate (Boniva®). Since they affect bone formation and stay in a person's bones after they've been taken, these drugs may pose a risk to the fetus. Therefore, doctors often advise women to wait until menopause before taking osteoporosis drugs.

When I was diagnosed with osteopenia, I felt that it was preferable to take preventive drugs before getting osteoporosis because:

◆ It's easier to prevent bone loss than to reverse it. If I waited until I had osteoporosis to take alendronate, it would be harder to make my bones resistant to breakage.

◆ The diagnosis occurred just before menopause when my periods were becoming irregular. The greatest potential for bone loss in a woman is typically just before menopause and during the first few years after menopause. After that, the percentage of yearly loss tends to diminish. Therefore, it made sense to take a preventive drug around menopause.

This logic has been valid for estrogen therapy. The Harvard Medical School Report entitled "Boosting Bone Strength" (p 7) states that estrogen therapy is most effective in retarding bone loss when started just after the onset of menopause, and "the earlier estrogen is initiated, the more pronounced its effects." On the other hand, estrogen treatment begun five or more years after menopause had little effect on risk, even when continued for longer than a decade.

◆ Bones must be strong to withstand all types of exercise, and exercise is essential for maintaining strong bones. I believed that drug therapy might help my back withstand the force of strength training, which in turn would make it stronger.

◆ I was physically able to take alendronate. Later, I might have gastro-intestinal problems or other conditions that would make it an unsuitable drug for me.

◆ I was financially able to pay for alendronate. I may not be able to afford it later on, especially if I were to need non-optional medications.

Another doctor that would probably have advised me to take medication is Harris H. McIlwain, MD, chairman of the Florida Osteoporosis Board. In his book, *Reversing Osteopenia*, he says "Very strong evidence exists that many fractures in postmenopausal women actually happen when bone mass is in the osteopenia range. Some studies show that many fractures (as many as 50% or more) actually happen when T-scores show osteopenia, not osteoporosis. . . . In our clinical practice we've found that if a woman has osteopenia plus other risk factors present, it is often a good idea to add medications as part of her fracture prevention program." (P. 102 & 103 of *Reversing Osteopenia* coauthored by Debra Fulghum Bruce, PhD)

In October 2004, the results of a follow-up study of one of the first alendronate clinical trials was presented (FIT, Fracture Intervention Trial). Women who had taken alendronate for five years were randomly given a placebo or more alendronate for the next five years. During that time, the number of fractures was the same for the two groups of women. These results indicate that unlike hormones, alendronate offers fracture protection even after it's stopped and it may not be necessary to take it after five years. In other words, alendronate appears to be most effective at decreasing fracture risk during the first five years it is taken. It remains to be seen if people who stop taking alendronate after five years will need to get booster doses of alendronate in order to have lifetime protection against bone loss.

Currently women entering menopause have two main options if their bone density reports show areas of low bone mass and natural methods are not preventing loss of bone:

1. To wait until they get osteoporosis to take bone-boosting drugs. Gaining back lost bone, however, will be difficult.

2. To avoid getting osteoporosis by taking bone drugs during the first few years after menopause, the time they are most apt to lose bone. Later, when their potential for bone loss levels off, they may choose to continue or stop the drug and just monitor their bone density. I think this preventive approach is the more desirable option.

In my case, the combination of drug therapy, strength training and a healthy diet including soy products was so effective at improving my bone density that I was able to reduce and discontinue the alendronate.

Why I've Never Taken Hormones

I've never had hormonal problems, so I've never taken hormones. However, the experience of a family friend, whom I will call Bertha, made me vow to never take hormones for the prevention of osteoporosis.

Bertha was about 80 when her doctor prescribed an estrogen plus progestin pill as a treatment for osteoporosis. Right after she started taking it, her breasts began to hurt. About six months later she had an abnormal mammogram, even though it had always been normal before. Shortly thereafter, Bertha fell, and profuse vaginal bleeding followed. To make sure she did not have cancer, Bertha had to undergo gynecological tests and follow-up mammograms. About a year later, she stopped taking hormones and all of her female organ problems disappeared.

When I mentioned to a friend what happened to Bertha, my friend told me she'd had a similar experience after starting to use wild yam cream, a progesterone ointment. Prior to applying the cream, her mammograms were normal. A few months after beginning the hormonal therapy, she had an abnormal mammogram. Instead of immediately getting a biopsy, she decided to stop using the progesterone cream; her mammograms returned to normal.

The US Surgeon General's 2004 *Bone Health & Osteoporosis* report (pp 230 & 231) says "The clear benefits of postmenopausal HT (hormone therapy) to the skeleton must be tempered by the other results from the WHI (Women's Health Initiative) trials, which were discontinued early because of the deleterious effects encountered. Both trials found an increased risk of stroke, cognitive impairment and deep vein thrombosis in the women taking HT. Breast cancer risk was increased in women taking the combined continuous therapy (E+P) during the 5.2 years of the study, a finding that is consistent with observational studies."

The Prempro® hormone website (www.prempro.com) states that using estrogens with or without progestins may increase your chances of getting heart attacks, strokes, breast cancer, blood clots and dementia. Hormones can be a godsend for women who have hormonal imbalances or who have had their ovaries surgically removed. However, when used to prevent osteoporosis, the risks for many women seem to outweigh the benefits.

"Natural" Hormones

Progesterone creams that are manufactured from plant compounds may help prevent bone loss, but no long-term, double-blind clinical trials have been done to test their effectiveness. One of these ointments, wild yam cream, is sometimes described by sellers as a safe and natural alternative to hormone replacement therapy. However, due to lack of research, we don't know if wild yam cream may have some of the same adverse risks as prescription hormones.

Out of curiosity, I read the leaflet that accompanied a tube of wild yam cream. It stated under "Considerations" that there have been reports of incidental spotting which may be associated with progesterone use, and that any persistent spotting or breakthrough bleeding should always be checked by a physician. It also said that natural progesterone can potentially increase thyroid activity.

In her book *Better Bones, Better Body,* nutritionist Susan Brown says, "Hormones, even 'natural' ones are powerful substances and should be given in the appropriate doses according to individual need. . . . Self administration of hormones or the prescription of hormone therapy without proper testing can create an even greater imbalance."

Don't assume that a product that's labeled as "natural" is safe and free of side effects. There are lots of natural plants, which are not safe such as poison ivy.

As a consumer writer about gems, I'm surprised that sellers of wild yam cream and other similar products are allowed to identify their products as natural. The ingredients of the tube of wild yam that I examined listed several different chemical ingredients, one of which happened to be extract of wild yam (Dioscorea villosa 3%).

In the gem trade, only a gemstone mined from the ground can be called natural. Even if a man-made ruby has the same chemical composition and structure as natural ruby, if it was created in a laboratory, the stone must be described by terms such as synthetic, man-made, lab-grown, lab-created, etc. It cannot be called a natural ruby. If a stone doesn't have the same chemical composition as ruby but is used to simulate ruby, then it's an imitation ruby.

When you buy "natural" products, look at the ingredients to determine how natural they are. The word "natural" is an effective marketing term, but don't be misled by it. If you'd like to get some beneficial plant hormones that are natural, then drink soy milk or eat soy foods, which contain plant estrogens. Unfortunately, you can't get similar benefits by eating wild Mexican yams or by spreading mashed yams on your body. They must be put through a lengthy conversion process in a chemistry lab in order to manufacture progesterone; the human body cannot achieve the conversion by itself.

Some Criticisms and Advantages of Osteoporosis Drugs

Fosamax® (alendronate) is the most frequently criticized bone drug because it is the most widely used. The strongest attacks I've seen against alendronate have been from doctors who sell "natural" hormones, bone building supplements, and other pills, foods or equipment that are supposed to prevent or cure osteoporosis. In this section, I list their three main objections to alendronate and explain why their arguments didn't convince me to stop taking it and use their products instead. These arguments can also be used against similar drugs (bisphosphonates) such as Actonel (risedronate) and Boniva (ibandronate). Included in this section is a chart listing advantages and disadvantages of osteoporosis drugs.

◆ **Alendronate can cause gastrointestinal problems** such as ulcers of the esophagus, heartburn, diarrhea, and abdominal pain. Even the alendronate website, www.Fosamax.com, acknowledges these side effects. One doctor indicated in a report that the effects are so severe some people have to be rushed to hospitals because of bleeding ulcers, but he sells bone boosting products.

Another doctor selling "miracle" bone-building pills said that the side effects of Fosamax are so bad that you have to wait at least a half hour after you take it to eat food or drink coffee. That's inaccurate. The reason you have to wait to eat is so that the alendronate can be absorbed into your system. Since food and beverages including mineral water reduce the absorption of alendronate, you must take it in the morning on an empty stomach with a glass of distilled water. Then you must sit upright or stand until you have food. This is true, too, of risedronate and ibandronate. Since ibandronate is only taken once a month, and risedronate and alendronate are usually taken once a week, this regimen is not much of an inconvenience.

If you lie down before you eat, this could increase the risk of esophageal irritation and ulcers. Likewise, if you have side effects and continue taking the drugs, the side effects could get worse.

I've never noticed any side effects from alendronate and neither have most of the people I've interviewed. However, one lady I met got a stomach ache the first time she tried alendronate, so she never took any more, and she never had any more problems. Another had bone pains, which ceased when she stopped the drug.

One other woman got a stomach ulcer about three years after she started taking it. She had forgotten the possible side effects of alendronate and had ignored her diarrhea and stomach pain for several months until the ulcer was discovered. She stopped taking the drug even though it had helped her bone density, but it took a few months for the ulcer to heal. The moral of the story?—Stop taking drugs like alendronate, risedronate, or ibandronate if you have stomach pain or gastrointestinal problems, and call your doctor. People who take aspirin or other drugs that can irritate the stomach are more likely to have side effects than people who take no such medications. Incidentally, drugs like alendronate can also be administered intravenously if people have stomach or esophagus problems.

On page 206 of her book *What Your Doctor May Not Tell You about Osteoporosis,* Dr. Cosman states that the gastrointestinal side effects of alendronate are reduced substantially when taking it once a week instead of daily. "This is because the lining of the esophagus replaces itself every day or two, so that if there is any irritation, it is repaired and there is no further irritation."

One must always weigh the risks and benefits before starting any drug therapy program. For example, if I hadn't taken alendronate, I believe I would have had a greater risk of fracture and bone loss. On the other hand, taking the drug could have led to gastrointestinal problems. I'd rather get an ulcer than break a bone or suffer the circulatory and female-organ side effects of hormones. Consequently, I followed my doctor's advice and took alendronate. When my bone density reversed its downward trend and reached more normal levels, I didn't think I needed the drug. However, I can always take it again if necessary.

◆ **Alendronate may cause bones to be brittle or abnormal.** Randomized, controlled trials have shown that alendronate reduces bone fractures, suggesting that it doesn't make bones brittle.

Sidney Bonnick, MD, medical director of the Clinical Research Center of North Texas, says that "in the dose that we use to prevent or treat osteoporosis, it [alendronate] simply does not cause the bone to become abnormal" (p 163 of her book *The Osteoporosis Handbook).* Bone biopsies of people on alendronate have been compared to those of people not taking the drug to determine that it's safe.

A recent study of 818 elderly women funded by the National Institute of Aging found that women taking alendronate or estrogen had significantly fewer bone abnormalities associated with severe knee osteoarthritis (e.g., bone spurs, bone thickening under the cartilage and bone marrow edema-like lesions) than women not taking the medication. MRI's were used to assess the prevalence of bone abnormalities. Women taking alendronate also had less knee pain. The study found, too, that estrogen may protect against the development of bone abnormalities associated with knee osteoarthritis. (November 2004 issue of *Arthritis & Rheumatism*)

If alendronate were taken to excess, it could have a negative effect on the bones and the body. This is also true of calcium. (See Chapters 8 and 9.)

◆ **We don't know the long-term effects of alendronate**. This is true. But we do know the effects of it on women who have taken it for ten years. Alendronate has been able to prevent bone loss and reduce fractures without causing bone abnormalities or serious side effects during the ten-year period. Patients who are uncomfortable about potential long-term effects can take the drug for shorter periods of time.

Table 11.1 Osteoporosis Medications

Drug Class & Names	Advantages	Disadvantages
Bisphosphonates Actonel® (risedronate) Boniva® (ibandronate) Fosamax® (alendronate) Didrocal® (etidronate) not used in US for osteoporosis	Slow down the bone- eroding cells; increase bone density and reduce fractures. Boniva has only been shown to reduce the risk of spine fractures.	Risk of ulcers and gastrointestinal side effects. May cause bone or muscular pain. Must be taken on an empty stomach while upright.
SERM's (Selective Estrogen Receptor Modulators) Evista® (raloxifene)	Act like the hormone estrogen in the bones. Increase bone density and reduce risk of spine fractures.	Risk of blood clots. May cause hot flashes, leg cramps, abdominal pain. No significant reduction in non-vertebral fractures has been reported.
Estrogen and/or progestin estrogen: Cenestin, Estrace, Premarin, Ogen, Ortho-Est. estrogen patch: Alora, Climara, Estraderm, Vivelle progestin: Provera estrogen + progestin: Femhrt, Activella,, Prefest, Prempro, Premphase	Increases bone density and reduces the risk of spine and hip fractures. Relieves menopausal symptoms.	Risk of blood clots, stroke, breast cancer, gallbladder disease, endometrial cancer, cardiovascular disease, depression, weight gain and dementia.
Hormonal bone resorption **inhibitor** (a hormone produced in the thyroid) Calcitonin: Miacalcin® (a nasal spray)	Slows down the bone- eroding cells (osteoclasts) helping prevent bone loss. Increases bone density slightly and reduces risk of spinal fractures.	May cause nasal ulcers, mild flu-like symptoms; not as effective as bisphos- phonates at increasing bone density. Not shown to reduce risk of hip fractures.
Bone formation agent — **parathyroid hormone** Forteo® (teriparatide) only for people with osteoporosis and at high risk of fracture	Activates the bone- building cells thereby generating new cells. Increases bone density and reduces risk of fractures.	Risk of bone cancer. A lot more expensive than other osteoporosis drugs, must be given by injection. May cause dizziness, nausea and leg cramps.
Bone formation agent Protelos® (strontium ranelate) released to the European market in 2004. Not available in North America	Stops breakdown of bone and stimulates bone growth; first treatment that performs both functions. Reduces the risk of hip and spine fractures.	Risk of blood clots. May cause mild nausea and diarrhea; taken daily at bedtime at least two hours after eating.

Sources: *PDR Monthly Prescribing Guide, Bone Health and Osteoporosis*, www.nof.org, www.nos.org.uk/public.asp, www.osteofound.org, and www.osteoporosis.ca

Most of this chapter focused on alendronate because I have experience using it. Since I'm not a doctor and I haven't taken any other osteoporosis drugs, I haven't written much about them. However, on the preceding page, I have summarized the benefits and drawbacks of the various osteoporosis medications. Talk with your physician about the different drug options. Free information about the different osteoporosis medications can be found on the following pharmaceutical and osteoporosis organization websites:

www.nof.org — National Osteoporosis Foundation (USA)
www.nos.org.uk/public.asp — National Osteoporosis Society (UK)
www.osteofound.org — International Osteoporosis Foundation
www.osteoporosis.ca — Osteoporosis Society of Canada
www.osteoporosis.ca — Osteoporosis Society of Canada
www.actonel.com
www.evista.com
www.forteo.com
www.fosamax.com
www.calcitonin.com
www.myboniva.com
www.servier.com/pro/identification.asp (site for Protelos based in France)
www.servier.co.uk/patients/osteoporosis.asp (based in UK)

If you decide to use an osteoporosis drug, don't use it as an excuse for inactivity. It's just as important to exercise, eat healthy food and get adequate calcium, vitamin D, magnesium and other nutrients when you are taking an osteoporosis medication as when you are not.

12

Vibrating Platform Therapy

Vibrating platform therapy is a new method of preventing osteoporosis that requires no drugs. It involves standing on a vibrating platform about the size of a bathroom scale for 10–20 minutes a day. You can read or watch TV at the same time. The subtle vibrations mimic the tiny contractions of muscle cells, thereby exerting small stresses on the bone that stimulate bone-building cells.

This new therapy is the result of over two decades of research into finding ways to prevent bone loss in astronauts. Even though they get proper nutrition, exercise and calcium, astronauts lose bone during prolonged exposure to weightlessness (1%–2% per month on average). This is how we learned about the importance of weight bearing and resistance activities for the prevention of osteoporosis. (www.science.nasa.gov)

Research on vibration therapy has been funded in part by NASA, the National Institutes of Health, the US Army, and the Russian government. Experiments were first conducted on animals such as turkeys, sheep and rats. The results have shown that tiny, barely perceptible vibrations can prevent bone loss, increase bone mass and build muscle in these animals. The challenge was to find a safe and effective vibrational frequency and intensity for humans.

The vibrating platform shown in figure 12.1 transmits high-frequency, low-intensity vibrations and has proved to be both safe and effective at preventing bone loss.

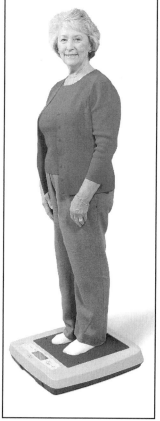

Fig. 12.1 A Juvent platform for preventing bone loss.
Photo courtesy Juvent, Inc.

The inventors of the technology are Drs. Kenneth McLeod and Clinton Rubin, both from the State University of New York (SUNY). Juvent licenses their patents and has many patents of its own on the device. During the fall of 2005, the vibrating platform was introduced to the market in Australia, New Zealand, the United Kingdom, Ireland, Germany, and Austria. As of January 2006, the FDA in the United States was still considering it for approval. Check the Juvent website, www.juvent.com, to find out if and when it will be available in your area. This website also has examples of published research studies on vibrating plate therapy. You can find them by clicking on "scientific information." NASA recently selected the Juvent technology for use on the International Space Station in 2007.

Promising Results for Lay People

The benefits of vibrating platform therapy are not limited to astronauts. Studies have been conducted on disabled children with low bone density, adolescent girls, and postmenopausal and premenopausal women with low bone density. The results are promising. For example, a randomized, double-blind study on 70 postmenopausal women showed that after a year, the women using a real vibrating platform had an average 2%–3% advantage over the placebo group in preventing bone loss at the lumbar spine and hip. The better the compliance to the therapy, the better the results. Lighter-weight people tended to benefit the most. Subjects who routinely engaged in high impact activity or resistance training were excluded from the study. (*Journal of Bone & Mineral Research*, Vol. 19, No. 3, March 2004, pp 343–351).

In another clinical trial on children with cerebral palsy, there was an 11% increase in density in the tibia bone after six months of treatment, in contrast to a 6% loss of bone density in children standing on placebo devices (*Journal of Bone & Mineral Research*, Vol. 19, No. 3, March 2004, pp 360–369).

Animal research suggests that vibration therapy improves both strength (resistance to fracture) as well as bone density. In one study, bone from sheep who had stood with their hind limbs on a vibrating plate (30 Hz, 0.3g) was compared to that of sheep who had stood on an inactive plate. During the course of a year, both groups of adult female sheep spent 20 minutes per day, five days per week on the plate. The rest of the time they were allowed to freely roam on pasture. After the test, the sheep were euthanized, and a cube of trabecular bone from their upper left femora underwent analysis and simulated compression tests. The results showed that the bone of the vibrated sheep was both stiffer (12%) and stronger

(27%), including in the two off axis-directions that were measured. (*Annals of Biomedical Engineering*, Vol. 31, pp 12–20, 2003.)

Making Vibration Therapy Safe

In an attempt to prevent osteoporosis, people may go overboard on vibration therapy and use devices with vibrations that are so strong they are unsafe for the body. Considerable research has been done on the effect of vibrations on workers who use jackhammers, tractors and other similar types of industrial equipment. The results have shown that long-term exposure to whole body vibration can cause permanent damage to the nerves, muscles, joints, back, heart and circulatory system.

Consequently, medical boards and government agencies have been cautious about authorizing vibration therapy for osteoporosis. The vibrations must fall within the limits set by the International Organization for Standardization (ISO) and the U.S. Occupational Safety and Health Administration (OSHA).

Realizing the potential risks of vibration therapy, the Juvent company worked on designing a platform with the smallest types of vibrations necessary for stimulating bone growth. The vibrations of the Juvent are so subtle (0.3 g's at 32 to 37 Hertz) that users hardly feel them. In addition, during the first eleven seconds of motion on the platform, the device's processor selects the most efficient and safe frequency for the user.

According to Juvent, a 20-minute session per day can help increase bone density by an average of 1%–2% a year. A digital display on the Juvent device automatically displays the time remaining in treatment and the total number of treatments. Vibrating platform therapy should not be used by people with conditions in which an increase in fluid to the heart may be detrimental, e.g., congestive heart failure. Always consult your doctor before undertaking medical treatment.

Vibrating platform therapy can be done at home or at a clinic or doctor's office. It should not be used as a substitute for exercise. Besides helping to prevent bone loss, exercise improves balance and strengthens your muscles and heart. The best gains in bone mass usually occur when osteoporosis therapies are combined with exercise and good nutrition.

13

Understanding Density Reports

In 1998, I walked into a drugstore that was offering bone density finger tests for $25. Since I was 50 and my mother had a broken hip, I decided to have the test done. The tester gave me a one-page printout of the report, showing an x-ray type image of my finger, a reference graph of the results, and numerical tables. She then said the results indicated my bone density was above that of the average young adult. Here are some of the results from the report I received:

Bad*	0.594 g/cm^2		
T-score	+1.2	+1.2	Relative to a young healthy adult
Z-score	+1.3	+1.3	Age-matched BMD
Analysis	High BMD		Based on WHO guidelines

*BMD: Bone mineral density. It tells how much mineralized bone tissue is packed into a square centimeter of bone.

T-score Legend

Above 1	High bone mineral density
Between 1 and -1	Normal
Between -1 and -2.5	Osteopenia (low bone mass)
-2.5 and below	Osteoporosis

Since my finger scores were relatively high, I was confident after the test that I would never have to be concerned about osteoporosis. I figured I could even lose bone mass and still be in the normal range.

A year after my finger test, I took my mother to a testing center for a bone density test of her hip and spine. The doctor who analyzed the results said my mother had severe osteoporosis and showed us the images of her spine and hip. Then he outlined various treatment options and preventive measures, which my mother later discussed with her regular physician.

Afterwards, he told me that her diagnosis meant that I was at risk of getting osteoporosis. When I mentioned the high T-score of my finger test, he said it could be a misleading indicator and that I should have my spine and hip tested because they were more susceptible to fractures. Then he suggested that I tell my doctor about my mother's results and get a more diagnostic test.

If this density center had not stressed the importance of spine and hip density tests, I doubt I would have been willing to pay for one, and I would not have alerted my doctor to my mother's history of osteoporosis. Instead, I got tested and established baseline densities of my spine and hip. This allowed me to learn 2 ½ years later that my hip density was declining significantly, even before menopause. I also found out that I had low bone mass in my spine. Because of this information, I was able to take preventive measures against osteoporosis in time to avert it.

What is a T-score?

On bone density reports, a T-score is a statistical measure of how far the bone density deviates from that of an average healthy young adult. In other words, **a T-score is a number that compares your bone density to that of a young adult**. "The term "T-score" is considered as one word; the horizontal line between "T" and "score" is a hyphen, not a minus sign.

If the T-score is 0.0 on a density report, this means the bone mineral density (BMD) is the same as that of the average young adult.

If the T-score is 1.0, the bone density is about 10-12 percent above that of the average young adult. Usually, 1 SD equals a 10–12 percent change in bone density. Statistically speaking, a T-score of 1.0 means the BMD is one standard deviation (SD) above the norm.

If the T-score is -1.0, the bone density is 1 standard deviation *below* that of the average young adult. The lower the T-score, the higher your fracture risk.

The World Health Organization (WHO) uses T-scores to define osteoporosis and osteopenia as follows:

◆ **Normal: T-score at or above -1.0.**

◆ **Osteopenia** (low bone mass or low bone density): **T-score between -1 and -2.5.** This may sound like a serious diagnosis, but it usually isn't. Felicia Cosman, MD, clinical director of the National Osteoporosis

Foundation, says that fracture risk in this range is generally low, and that most women in their sixties have bone density values in the osteopenic range or below.(p 123 of *What Your Doctor May Not Tell You about Osteoporosis)*

A diagnosis of osteopenia is mainly a warning to take action against getting osteoporosis. In some women, though, who have other important risk factors, such as previous fracture or a strong family history of fractures, or with certain underlying diseases, osteopenia may have more important implications.

◆ **Osteoporosis**: **T-score at or below -2.5**. A score in this range does not mean you will break a bone if you fall; it just means that you have a higher fracture risk than people with normal bone mass. The lower the score the higher the risk.

◆ **Severe (established) osteoporosis**: T-score at or below -2.5 and one or more osteoporotic fractures have occurred.

The above definitions apply only when a young healthy Caucasian woman reference database is used to determine T-scores.

Often next to the T-score, a percentage figure is included. For example, if the T-score of the total left hip is -0.1, then "99%" may be placed next to the score. This figure means that the patient has 99% of the bone density of a healthy young adult.

What is a Z-Score?

A Z-score is a statistical measure that compares your BMD to that of other people of the same age and gender. Depending on the manufacturer of the device, race and body size may also be factored into the comparison.

The Z-score is not used to diagnose osteoporosis; it's used to determine how normal or abnormal your bone density is for your age. If the Z-score is below -1.5, this suggests that something other than aging or menopause might be causing abnormal bone loss. If the cause can be identified and treated, the bone loss can often be slowed or stopped.

What's More Important: The T-score or the Z-score?

The T-score is more important because it's the score used for diagnosis. Nevertheless, the Z-score is helpful for indicating how you measure up to your age group and for alerting you to check for underlying causes of bone loss other than age or menopause.

If your goal is to feel good about yourself, then pay more attention to the Z-score. If your goal is to prevent osteoporosis and avoid fractures, then focus on improving or maintaining your T-scores—in other words your current bone mass.

When I'm eighty, I'd rather have the bone density of a healthy young adult or a middle-aged person than that of the average eighty-year-old woman. Therefore it's the T-score that I care about most.

What's the Difference Between the T-Score and BMD?

A T-score is a statistical number that tells how far your bone density deviates from that of an average young adult. BMD, the acronym for bone mineral density, is the amount of mineral in a given volume of bone. A BMD numerical value indicates the density of a specified area of your skeleton, without any reference to another person.

The T-score is used for diagnosing osteoporosis and osteopenia, whereas the BMD is used for determining the percentage of your bone loss or gain between tests. For example, if 1.000 is the BMD of your total hip in your first density test and 0.900 is the BMD of your total hip two years later, this means your total hip data showed a 10% bone loss in two years.

14

Bone Density Testing

Nowadays, you don't have to wait until you break a bone to find out if you have osteoporosis. You can have your bone density measured by a variety of types of machines.

Types of Bone Density Tests

Peripheral dual energy x-ray absorptiometry (pDXA). This measures only the peripheral sites of the body such as the finger, wrist and heel. It's one of the least expensive types of density tests, costing as little as $25.

Dual energy x-ray absorptiometry (DXA or DEXA). Currently the preferred type of bone density test, DXA is typically used to measure the spine and hip, but it can also measure the total body or individual peripheral sites. Like the pDXA, the radiation exposure is minimal— less than 1/10 of a chest X-ray (sometimes described as the same amount of radiation as you might get during an international flight). As a result, the technician can remain in the room with you during the test. Specifics on the amount of radiation exposure of various types of tests are given on page 10 of the National Osteoporosis Foundation Brochure "How Strong are Your Bones."

The DXA test is painless and normally takes less than twenty minutes. A scanner moves back and forth over your body while you lie on a padded scanning table. The price of a DXA test of the spine and hip typically ranges from $125 to $180.

Single energy x-ray absorptiometry (SXA). Low priced and portable, it measures bone density in the wrist or heel. This has been replaced by DXA tests, which are more accurate and can check the spine and hip bones.

Quantitative ultrasound (QUS). Used to measure bone density of the heel, shin bone and kneecap, QUS involves no radiation and is widely used as a low-cost screening tool. It measures the reflection of sound waves. The denser your bone, the faster sound waves are reflected back to the machine.

Radiographic absorptiometry (RA) This low-priced procedure uses ordinary x-rays and an aluminum wedge to calculate bone density.

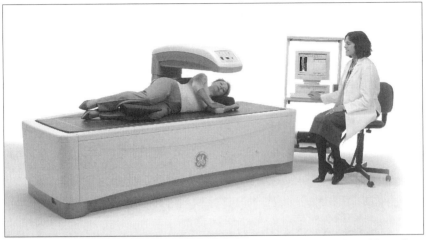

Fig. 14.1 A DXA densitometer (GE Prodigy™ Advance) and monitor. *Photo from GE Healthcare.*

Quantitative computed tomography (QCT). Primarily used in research for measuring the density of the spine, QCT provides detailed, three-dimensional images of the skeleton. It's more expensive and uses much more radiation than DXA tests.

Peripheral QCT (pQCT). Seldom used, this is an adaptation of QCT, which provides an accurate and less costly way of measuring trabecular and cortical bone in the forearm.

Heel Tests Versus DXA Spine and Hip Tests

Heel tests are a cost-effective way to screen for fracture risk. However, they only measure the heel; they don't tell you the density of your spine and hip, which can be significantly lower. Consequently, heel tests may give people a false sense of security about their bone health.

I had an opportunity to get an ultrasound heel test after I'd already had DXA tests. Out of curiosity, I decided to have the test done. I received a score of +0.4. The summary report interpreted this score to mean that I'm at low risk for bone diminishment. I knew that wasn't true, however; even before menopause, my hip bone density had decreased over 7% during a 2 ½-year period. The heels of my feet get a lot of direct bone-boosting impact from walking and running, so it's understandable that I have a high heel score. Like my finger test, the heel test gave misleading results, which could have kept me from taking preventive measures had I not had prior DXA tests of the spine and hip.

When the heel results are low, the test offers two main benefits—it can alert you about your risk of osteoporosis, and it may enable you to have the cost of a DXA test paid for by an insurance company or government health plan. Follow-up and comparative tests should be done on DXA densitometers. They're more accurate and complete; and unlike QCT tests, use little radiation.

How Accurate are Bone Density Tests?

You should expect about a 1–2 percent margin of error for bone density tests done on the newer models of DXA machines. Precision studies of these newer models have reported values ranging from 0.9 percent to 2.3 percent (*Bone Densitometry for Technologists* by Sydney Bonnick, MD, p 43). This is an improvement over densitometers produced in the 1990's.

If the test is repeated on a different machine, the margin of error can be as high as 10 percent because the types of filters and/or systems used to measure the bone density may be different. Therefore, **have follow-up tests done on the same densitometer as the first test,** when possible. Otherwise the results may cause you to make false conclusions.

The margin of error on different densitometers is usually lower if the machines are from the same manufacturer and if they were purchased after 2000. Older machines tend to show more variation.

When interpreting your T-scores and comparing them to those of friends and relatives keep in mind the following:

◆ **The reference databases for the T-scores may vary**. T-scores are based on the bone density of the average healthy young adult. The ages of the subjects can range anywhere from 20–40 years, but the cutoff points for the ages vary from one data base to another; one cutoff point is from 20–29 years. The percentage of athletic women in the database may also vary, and this will affect the average BMD values of the group.

Since manufacturers of densitometers do not all use the same database, the significance of their T-scores may vary. This is another reason why you should do repeat tests on the same densitometer.

◆ **Total spine and hip scores can be misleading**. Often as people age, their spine undergoes arthritic changes, which causes some vertebrae to have a much higher density than the other vertebrae. Knowledgeable testing centers may exclude the falsely elevated vertebrae when averaging the densities of the lumbar vertebrae. Felicia Cosman, MD, clinical director of the National Osteoporosis Foundation, says that

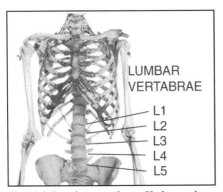

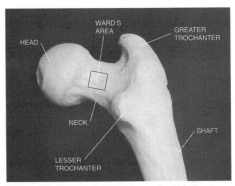

Fig 14.2 Lumbar vertebrae. *Skeleton photo*   **Fig. 14.3** Femoral hip. *Photo by Ed Newton.*
courtesy of www.skullsunlimited.com.

many times she's seen patients who have had their bone densities mis-interpreted. This is because a person's total-spine T-score can be normal if the density of one or two of the bones is substantially falsely elevated (p. 114 of *What Your Doctor May Not Tell you about Osteoporosis*).

Arthritic changes seldom affect the bone density of the hip. Nevertheless total hip scores can also be misleading. If, for example, the density of the neck of your hip is lower than average, but the density of the shaft is higher than normal, your total hip score may average out to be normal. Yet your hip still could be at risk for breakage at the neck, a common fracture site. Therefore, don't assume that your bones are fine if your total hip and spine T-scores are in the normal range.

According to World Health Organization guidelines, the diagnosis should be based on the worst of the T-scores because the site with the lowest bone density is at the highest risk for fracture.

The November 2003 Official Positions of the International Society for Clinical Densitometry (ISCD) recommended that test centers choose the lowest of the T-scores among the femoral neck, total hip, greater trochanter and lumbar spine. In their September 2005 Official Positions, the trochanter is no longer included as a site to be used for diagnosis (www.iscd.org). Nevertheless, it's still important to consider the density of the trochanteric region because it's a common site for hip fractures.

◆ **The definition of the total lumbar spine score can vary.** Some test centers usually base their spine T-score on the average of the 1st to 4th lumbar vertebrae, other centers on the 2nd to 4th lumbar vertebrae, or 2nd and 3rd. In addition, radiologists may exclude vertebrae with falsely elevated T-scores when determining the average T-score of the spine.

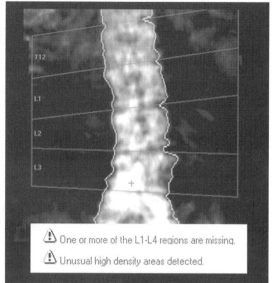

Fig 14.4 Notice the vertebra with the cross. The densitometer has placed the cross on it to indicate that the surrounding white background is an area of unusually high density. If this vertebra were included in the overall measurement of the lumbar spine, the T-score would probably be falsely elevated.

Besides showing density differences, DXA images like these provide clues about the alignment and structural integrity of the spine.

Photo from GE Healthcare.

The diagnosis can change depending on the vertebrae used to determine score. Hence, **when comparing overall spine T-scores, check the reports to find out how the scores were established.**

Despite the number of variables involved in determining bone density, accurate conclusions may be drawn. I've been tested on three different machines. Although some of the results have been significantly different, the reports came up with the same diagnosis of osteopenia, except in the spring of 2005 when my diagnosis changed to normal. That diagnosis was confirmed by another densitometer.

To assure that you reach accurate conclusions about your bone density and response to treatment, try to get retested on the same densitometer, and remember to ask for detailed written copies of your bone density reports. A summary report is not sufficient. You need to see the accompanying details of BMD's and T-scores of the various skeletal sites to correctly assess your bones and your progress and to design an effective exercise program for yourself.

Who Should be Tested?

The International Society of Clinical Densitometry (www.iscd.org) states that bone density tests should be performed on:

◆ Women 65 and older

◆ Postmenopausal women under 65 with risk factors

◆ Men 70 and older

◆ Adults with a fragility fracture

◆ Adults with a disease or condition associated with low bone mass or bone loss

◆ Adults taking medications associated with low bone mass or bone loss

◆ Anyone being considered for treatment

◆ Anyone being treated, to monitor progress

◆ Anyone not receiving therapy if evidence of bone loss would lead to treatment

Felicia Cosman, MD, medical director of the Clinical Research Center at Helen Hayes Hospital, suggests that women get a bone density test at menopause even in the absence of risk factors, whether or not the insurance is willing to pay. The risk factor list may miss identifying some women who are at high risk. (*What Your Doctor May Not Tell you About Osteoporosis*, p111)

In accordance with the guidelines of the ISCD, orthopedist Leon Root recommends that men seventy or older have a bone density test (p 36, *Beautiful Bones Without Hormones).* Men lose bone, too, but usually at a later age than women, unless they're taking steroids or other medications that can cause bone loss at an earlier age.

Women interested in establishing a baseline and avoiding hormone-related bone loss should consider having a DXA test when they start missing periods just before menopause. I had a significant amount of bone loss prior to menopause and so have other women (for examples, search "perimenopause and bone loss" on the Internet). I'm glad I didn't wait until menopause to take preventive measures against osteoporosis. It's difficult to regain lost bone.

Osteoporosis in Men

Even though osteoporosis is often considered an old-ladies' disease, males also lose bone with aging. However, they tend to get osteoporosis at an older age because they usually have a higher peak bone density than women, and they don't undergo the rapid bone loss associated with menopause.

Interestingly enough, middle-aged men can also get osteoporosis. The March 2004 issue of *Bicycling Magazine* reported about the relatively high incidence of osteopenia and osteoporosis in male cyclists. They cited a study in the August 2003 issue of *Osteoporosis International* stating that one 42-year-old cyclist who loved dairy products had borderline osteoporosis in his spine. Another 48-year-old cyclist had the bone density of someone twice his age. However, he drank one to two liters of cola per day.

The *Bicycling Magazine* article suggests that bone loss is more prevalent in cyclists for a number of reasons:

◆ **Cyclists engage in less weight-bearing activity than the average man**. Cycling's seated, off-the-ground position eliminates the impact on the legs that a runner or hiker gets. When cyclists don't ride, they usually rest.

◆ **Men engaged in intense training lose about 200 milligrams of calcium in sweat per hour**. The energy drinks they consume contain little, if any, calcium to replace what is lost. If they don't consume a lot of extra calcium from food and dairy products or supplements, the calcium they sweat out must come from their bones.

◆ **Cyclists are typically skinny**, and thin people are more likely to get osteoporosis than heavier people because of less body weight on the bones.

Cyclists are not the only men who get osteoporosis. Alcoholics and men who take steroids or antiseizure medication are especially susceptible. However, any man can end up with osteoporosis. I know a retired fire fighter who broke his arm at the age of 76 while traveling abroad. After he returned home, his endocrinologist gave him a density test and found he had osteoporosis. Now the former fireman is on alendronate (Fosamax).

Whether you're a man or a woman, your body needs good nutrition and bone-strengthening exercise. The earlier you take preventive measures against osteoporosis, the better.

How Often Should People Be Tested?

Many doctors recommend getting tested every two to three years after the first BMD test, except for older adults with above average T-scores; they may not need repeat testing. If a patient is starting osteoporosis drug therapy, doctors may suggest annual tests for the next couple of years to monitor the effectiveness of the treatment.

The International Society for Clinical Densitometry (ISCD) states that it's necessary to know the expected rate of change in bone density and the precision of the densitometer being used in order to determine the best time to repeat a bone density test. In some situations, such as starting high dose glucocorticoid therapy, a test may be done as often as every six months. If bone density is changing very little, then three to five years or longer may be appropriate. (www.iscd.org/Visitors/patient/index.cfm)

The US medicare system for seniors permits repeat BMD tests every two years. Likewise, many private insurance companies that cover BMD testing also require a two-year wait before they will pay for repeat tests.

When I started taking Fosamax, I didn't want to wait a year or two to find out if it was having an effect, so I requested a repeat test 6–7 months later, which I paid for. I was also interested in knowing the effectiveness of diet, exercise, and calcium intake. I began drug therapy around menopause, the time when women are especially likely to lose bone due to decreasing estrogen. I figured that even no change in my scores would be a positive indication, considering that bone loss at menopause may accelerate from about 3% up to 7% per year (*Beautiful Bones Without Hormones* by orthopedist Leon Root, p.7, and *Osteoporosis Handbook* by Sydney Lou Bonnick, MD, p 43).

I was surprised when the repeat test on the same densitometer showed a 3.4% increase in my total hip BMD. The spine (L2–L3) BMD had an insignificant 1.8% increase. These changes occurred in a seven-month period during which my bone density would normally be decreasing. A later test showed even higher increases within a period of six months— for example, a 5.8% increase at the neck of the hip. See Chapter 17 for detailed tables of the results of my DXA bone density tests.

I was glad I repeated my DXA tests earlier than recommended because:

◆ Unexpected changes in my exercise habits have occurred. Having tests at more frequent intervals has allowed me to monitor the effects of these changes better and determine the most beneficial exercise for me.

◆ Getting frequent reminders of decreases in bone density motivated me to make a lot of the positive changes that I wouldn't have made otherwise. These changes helped reverse the downward trend of my bone densities and bring them to more normal levels.

◆ Frequent testing helped determine when it was appropriate to stop drug therapy. I don't want to take medication unless I need it. The money saved from unnecessary drug costs can more than pay for DXA tests. Testing will also determine if I need to resume drug therapy.

Overall, my DXA reports have given me objective clinical evidence as to how Fosamax and different types of exercise have affected my bone density. I would rather base my choice of treatment on this type of evidence than on advertising hype or only on research studies that test people with different lifestyles than mine. I know all the diet, health and exercise variables involved in the results of my tests, but I don't know those of research subjects. Considering all I've learned, I'm glad I've had several tests, and I believe my money has been well spent.

Contrasting Experiences with Bone Density Testing

During my first two encounters with bone density testing, the results were discussed at the time of the test and preventive advice was given. (My first experience was a finger test at a pharmacy and the second one involved my mother's spine and hip test at a place I'll call Test Center B.)

Later, when I had a physical, I got a referral from my doctor for a DXA hip and spine test. An imaging center performed the test, but did not discuss the results with me or offer preventive advice. About two weeks later, the nurse from my doctor's office called and said my hip density was in the normal range, but my spine was borderline low. I was advised to make sure I was getting 1200–1500 mg of calcium per day and daily exercise.

During a discussion on DXA tests, a friend of mine in France told me she got the results of her exam about thirty minutes after the test. A medical professional at the center gave her a copy of the five-page report, explained it to her and gave her tips on preventing osteoporosis. A copy of the report was sent to her doctor.

I wondered if other DXA testing centers in America gave patients as much information as Test Center B, the pharmacy, and the French test center; so I started to ask people throughout the United States about their experiences at testing centers. I interviewed friends, relatives, business associates, and other people at conventions, social events and on planes.

Results of my Interviews about Bone Density Centers

I was surprised to learn that the majority of the people I interviewed did not get preventive advice or any test results at their DXA test centers, and many did not have an opportunity to discuss the results with their doctor afterwards. If the people got immediate information, it was often because the test was done in a doctor's office instead of at an imaging center.

Of the people I interviewed who had asked for written copies of their results, the reports were often summary reports of their average spine and hip densities; they seldom included the scores of the individual vertebrae or of the relevant parts of the hip. A few people, however, did get detailed reports; and one person who had been part of an osteoporosis study also received images of her entire spine and hip.

The people who discussed their DXA results at the test center and/or in a face-to-face discussion with their doctor were the ones most likely to take constructive steps to prevent osteoporosis after the test. Those who never received the results or who only got the results via phone seldom made any changes in their behavior, even when they had a diagnosis of osteopenia or osteoporosis. In my case, I saw my doctor when I went to get the written results of my second DXA test. The direct discussion and free drug samples encouraged me to start taking Fosamax and to add soy foods to my diet.

Are Bone Density Tests Worthwhile?

Insurance companies, government agencies, medical researchers and doctors often debate the value of bone density tests. Controversy exists as to whether or not bone density tests prevent fractures.

There is a straightforward answer. Bone density tests by themselves do not prevent fractures. It's what you do with the results of the tests that can determine their value. If DXA technologists do not give patients the results or preventive advice, the test may be of little value because many patients never discuss the results or osteoporosis prevention with their doctors.

During my interviews with people about their DXA test experiences, I learned that patients get the following types of feedback about their results:

1 Sometimes none—neither from the test center nor their doctor.
2 Often only a diagnosis of normal, osteopenia or osteoporosis, and that may be given by a nurse or secretary in the doctor's office.
3 Sometimes the overall T-scores of their spine and hip along with the diagnosis.
4 Occasionally a verbal explanation of their T-scores and their diagnosis, along with an opportunity to view their spine and hip on the monitor.
5 In addition to the #4 feedback, occasionally a copy of their bone density report, including the summary report, the T-scores and BMD's of the individual sites measured (the ancillary results), and images of the lumbar spine and hip(s).

Some people ignore the individual T-scores because they think that bone loss is only systemic. They only want to know an overall diagnosis. The details are also important because **bone loss and gain can be localized or systemic.** The classic illustration of this is the contrasting densities of a tennis player's right and left arm. The playing arm consistently has a higher density, and the more it is used, the higher the density tends to be. On the other hand, if an arm is paralyzed or gets little use, it can lose density.

To emphasize this point, I'll repeat a quote from the chapter on exercise.

Bone adapts its structure to become denser and stronger or weaker depending on functional demands. Adaptation from exercise and mechanical stimuli is local, unlike pharmacologic intervention, which systemically bathes the entire skeleton (and all other tissues) with a drug. *(Clinton T. Rubin, PhD, Professor and Chair, Department of Biomedical Engineering, State University of New York at Stony Brook)*

Learning that bone loss can be either systemic or localized helped me understand why my spine and hips had wide variations in densities and T-scores (the numbers that compare my bone density to that of a young adult). After analyzing my reports, I realized that the skeletal areas that were exercised most and subjected to the most stress had the highest T-scores.

For example, my fourth lumbar vertebra (L4) has had T-scores above $+1.0$, and the spine images indicated that the area between L4 and L5 was showing wear. This area was getting a lot of stress both from lower back exercises, bending, and my daily activities. On the other hand, my first lumbar vertebra (L1), which gets a lot less exercise, has had T-scores below -1.3. In addition, the DXA spine image indicates that the density of the vertebra above L1 is even lower.

If you have this type of information, you can pass it along to training professionals at your gym. I did, and this led them to focus training sessions more on my mid and upper back and avoid exercises that can cause additional wear to my lower lumbar spine. When designing an exercise program to meet your specific needs, T-scores of individual sites can often be more useful than T-scores that have been averaged or cover a broad area.

Knowing the T-scores of individual sites can also be more motivating than just knowing a general T-score. For example, it was the T-scores and declining density of my first lumbar vertebra that prompted me to take up strength training. I'm grateful that my second test center had a special note on the report about the lower density of this area.

If the medical profession and insurance industry would like to make bone density testing as worthwhile as possible, they should encourage all DXA testing centers to discuss the test results with patients and give them preventive advice. This concept is developed further in the next chapter.

If *you* would like to make DXA testing as worthwhile as possible, try to schedule the exam about a month before you see your doctor for a physical and ask for a detailed written copy of your report. If you read it before your doctor's appointment, you'll be better prepared to discuss what course of action you should take. If you go to a testing center that will show you your results on the monitor and explain them to you, you'll be even more prepared for a constructive discussion with your doctor. The next chapter provides further tips on making the most of your DXA testing experience.

Measuring Bone Turnover With Blood & Urine Tests

Even though blood and urine tests cannot measure bone density, they can sometimes determine how fast bone is being broken down and restored. During the bone remodeling process, remnants of bone collagen and enzymes associated with bone turnover are released into the bloodstream and urine. The tests that measure these by-products of the remodeling cycle are called **bone marker tests** or **bone turnover tests**. They report what is happening to your bones the day of the test and can detect changes in bone turnover within two or three months. Bone density tests, on the other hand, report the results of long-term skeletal changes.

The advantages of bone turnover blood and urine tests are that they:

◆ Allow us to see changes in bone turnover more quickly than DXA tests.

◆ Help determine if medical treatment is working.

◆ May indicate if medical conditions or medications such as corticosteroids are causing significant bone loss.

◆ Usually cost less than DXA tests of the hip and spine.

The limitations of bone turnover tests are:

◆ They can't be used for diagnosing osteoporosis or osteopenia.

◆ They can't determine where you are losing bone in your body.

◆ The test results can vary depending on diet, time of day, and a woman's menstrual cycles, thereby limiting the usefulness of the tests. Repeat tests should be done at the same time of day as the first one, preferably in the morning after an overnight fast.

In summary, blood and urine tests are helpful for monitoring treatment and for detecting the underlying causes of osteoporosis, but they are not a substitute for bone density testing. It's best to use bone marker tests in conjunction with DXA tests; but in most cases, the DXA test will suffice.

For more information on bone marker blood and urine tests see:

Bone Health and Osteoporosis A Report of the Surgeon General. U.S. Public Health Service, pp 208–212, 2004

What Your Doctor May Not Tell You about Osteoporosis by Felicia Cosman, MD, pp 133–135, 2004

15

Side Benefits of Density Tests

S ome people think that bone density is measured only to determine if you need medication for osteoporosis, but that's just one purpose of getting tested. Even if you never plan to take osteoporosis drugs, bone density tests can be beneficial.

How Bone Density Tests Can Help You

◆ **DXA tests of the lumbar spine and hip(s) can show which areas of your body need more exercise.** Even though an overall diagnosis of osteopenia or osteoporosis is useful for recommending drug therapy, it's not adequate for designing an effective exercise program for your body. You should also find out the T-scores of the individual sites that were measured. These scores indicate how the bone densities of various areas of your hip and lumbar spine compare to that of a young adult. If some of the areas have low bone mass and others are in the normal range, it may be advisable to spend more time on exercises that target the areas with low density. Well-planned exercise can be more beneficial than random exercise.

◆ **DXA test scores and images can indicate the extent of your osteoporosis and which areas of your body may need modified types of exercise**. If you have osteoporosis, understanding the numerical data on your report can help you determine how serious your condition is. For example, a T-score of -2.6 in only the femoral neck would lead to a diagnosis of osteoporosis, but it's not as bad as having T-scores below -4.5 in both the hip and the spine. Don't be content with just a diagnosis. You should know the severity of your condition.

Even if the diagnosis is normal, it's helpful to know if you have T-scores close to low bone mass such as -0.9. If you know enough to compare data from test to test, you can also tell if you're gaining bone, losing bone or remaining stable.

If your T-scores are really low in a particular area, a therapist may recommend that you avoid certain exercises. For example, it may be best not to do forward bending exercises and poses when the lumbar spine density is exceptionally low. Even in cases of abnormally high spine density, forward bending exercises might be unwise if the images show too much wear of the lumbar discs. .

◆ **DXA tests can help spot potential alignment problems.** For example, a friend who sent me a copy of her density report had a left-hip T-score significantly greater than that of her right hip (one standard deviation). She didn't think much of it at the time, but a few months later she developed back problems and had to get X-rays and an MRI before undergoing therapy. Through her ordeal she learned that her right leg was shorter and required a lift. In essence, her density report predicted a problem with her right leg that needed correction. My friend just didn't realize it, and nobody mentioned it to her.

Figure 15.1 is an example of a hip alignment problem noticeable on DXA images. Some hip problems can be corrected with non surgical measures before they become serious.

The DXA lumbar spine image in the preceding chapter (page 109) illustrates a spine with alignment problems. Images like these require a minimal amount of radiation and can be especially helpful to orthopedists, chiropractors, and physical therapists.

◆ **DXA images may show fractures and areas of degeneration.** Even though DXA images are not as sharp and detailed as x-rays, they can help detect problems that might otherwise go unnoticed. Sometimes non surgical measures can be taken to prevent the problem from becoming critical.

If a serious problem is suggested by the DXA image, the area in question can be x-rayed. Primary-care physicians shouldn't be expected to notice compression fractures and areas of degeneration because they don't see the original DXA images on the monitor. They only get a printout of the image, which may just be a small positive version. Some report images are clearer than others. In addition, general practitioners don't normally have specialized training in radiology. However, radiologists or osteoporosis specialists who see the actual computer images may be able to spot problems other than areas of low density.

Dual energy x-ray absorptiometry (DXA) is cost-effective and uses little radiation. For less than $200, a DXA test can provide a wide variety of information including images of the spine and both hips. This can help us plan individualized exercise programs and detect osteoporosis and other conditions, which in turn can help prevent fractures, and serious back and hip problems. We should take full advantage of this technology.

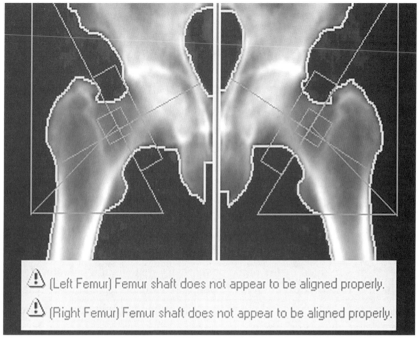

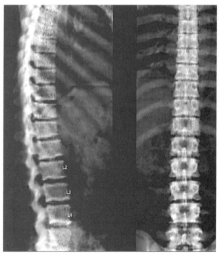

Fig. 15.1 Besides showing the areas of high density (white) and lowest density (black), DXA images like these give doctors information about the shape and angle of the bones and areas of possible degeneration. *Photo from GE Healthcare.*

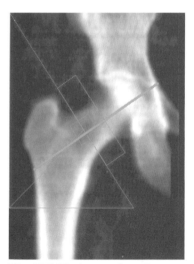

Fig. 15.2 Hip image of another person with a straighter shaft and longer femoral neck than that of the individual in Fig. 15.1. It's hypothesized that the shorter your hip axis length, the lower your risk of fracture, all other factors being equal. *Photo from GE Healthcare.*

Fig. 15.3 Front and side view DXA images of a spine. Normally only the lowest four or five vertebrae are shown on DXA reports. Images like these are especially helpful for orthopedists and chiropractors, and require a minimal amount of radiation. *Photo from GE Healthcare.*

Why Testing Centers Should Communicate with Patients

Medical technologists are often taught to refrain from discussing the results of tests with patients. The doctor who orders the test is supposed to be the person who answers the patient's questions about the results.

In theory, this sounds like a good approach. However, in the case of bone density tests, patients don't normally see their doctor right after the test. As much as a year may pass before they ever have an opportunity to discuss the test results face to face. If the patient has osteoporosis or osteopenia, the patient typically receives a phone call from the doctor's office with the diagnosis and recommendations for treatment. The message is sometimes relayed by the nurse or secretary instead of the doctor. If the results are normal, the patient may not receive any notice about the results.

In the previous chapter, I mentioned that when I was in France, a friend told me that she got a full written report of her test while at the density center. About a half hour after the test, a medical professional at the center brought her the report, explained it to her, answered her questions, and gave her preventive advice. I saw the report. It was five pages and had as much detailed data as my reports and included images of her spine and hip. Later, the center sent another copy of the report to her doctor, who would have determined the best type of treatment if it had been required.

In America, a few density testing centers offer preventive advice and answer patients' questions about their tests, but most do not. If a patient wants a written copy of their report, they usually must request it. (US law requires that test centers, hospitals and doctors give patients copies of their test results when asked). Other countries have similar laws.

Perhaps bone density centers assume that the patient's doctor should provide all of this information. During a physical, a doctor has to deal with all aspects of a patient's health, so the time allotted for talking about bone health is limited. Therefore, testing centers should share the responsibility of discussing test results and osteoporosis prevention.

It's possible to find a doctor who's a combination osteoporosis specialist, densitometrist, and radiologist. A density test conducted by this type of doctor may cost about the same as one done at an imaging center. However, you get more for your money—an opportunity to talk to a doctor, immediate feedback about your bones, and recommendations for treatment. Afterwards, you and your regular doctor can determine which treatment option is best.

It's best to be tested by an osteoporosis specialist. However, few doctors have densitometers and specialized training in bone density testing. If a patient has no access to an osteoporosis specialist, I think the French system of providing patients with information and preventive advice at the density test center is advantageous because:

◆ **Patients are better prepared to discuss treatment options** with their doctor if they understand what the numbers on their density tests mean.

◆ **It saves the doctor time**.

◆ **Bone density centers usually have more information than primary care physicians** about the patients DXA test results, and they're able to show the patient the images of their spine and hip on the computer monitor. It's hard for a general physician to be as knowledgeable about bone density tests as technologists who spend their entire workdays involved in bone density testing.

◆ **Repetition is important**. Even if the primary-care doctor has time to discuss the results and to give the patient preventive advice, it's good to hear it a second time. This reinforces the advice. Most people don't absorb and remember everything from the first explanation.

◆ **It can assure that patients learn their bone density test results from a trained professional.** In America, the nurse or the secretary in the doctor's office is sometimes the person who informs patients of their test results. Technologists at competent bone density testing centers often have more training in bone densitometry and osteoporosis prevention than general practitioners and internists.

◆ **It helps prevent errors of omission**. American doctors are so loaded with paperwork that they sometimes don't notice abnormal test results, or their patient loads are so heavy that they don't have time to discuss osteoporosis or the potential adverse effects of drugs.

For example, three endocrinologists in three different cities pre-scribed corticosteroid drugs for a friend of mine over a period of nine years, but not one of them told her that long-term use could lead to bone loss. It took her two years to wean herself off the drugs. Then when she had a bone density test, her general practitioner didn't notice until ten months later during an office visit that the results were abnormally low.

Bone density centers that discuss osteoporosis risk factors and that tell patients their results help prevent errors of omission.

As a consumer, you can prevent such errors by asking for copies of your reports and by doing research on drugs before you take them. You can get copies of your bone density reports either from the testing center or your doctor. Remember, in the United States and often elsewhere, they are required by law to give you a copy when asked.

Why Technologists May Not Discuss Test Results

One of the main reasons why many American technologists are not allowed to discuss density test results with patients is to avoid giving wrong or conflicting information. If a bone density test is given at an imaging center, the results must be interpreted by a radiologist, who then prepares a written report based on the data in the computer.

Even though the overall diagnosis is subject to change, the T-scores, Z-scores and bone mineral densities of the spine and hip are immediately calculated by the densitometer, and they don't change. It's hard to understand why many technologists are not allowed to at least give patients their numerical results. When pharmacies offer peripheral bone density tests, they tell you the T-scores and explain what the scores mean.

Like most people, I don't mind conflicting viewpoints or discrepancies in reports; after all medicine is not an exact science. However, if someone intentionally withholds my medical information from me or makes me wait a long time to get it, that upsets me.

Another reason why testing centers may not discuss test results is because they believe it's psychologically better for a doctor to tell patients bad news than for the technician to do so. I don't think this is a valid reason. Osteoporosis or osteopenia is not fatal like some diseases such as cancer can be; people don't die directly of osteoporosis. In addition, technologists can be taught to present data in a spirit of hope.

Even in more serious cases, it still can be helpful for a technologist to give patients information and let them look at the computer monitor. One example, unrelated to bone density testing, involves a carotid artery ultrasound test.

My mother's internist referred her to a vascular specialist after listening to her carotid arteries. The specialist mentioned surgery and sent her to an imaging center for an ultrasound of her carotids. I accompanied her to the center. During the test, the technologist told how much her arteries were blocked and he let us see them on the monitor.

The news was not good, but my mother was able to reflect upon it for a couple of days before her next appointment with the specialist. Even though she'd had a stroke before, she decided she did not want surgery. If she had a stroke or died as a result, she figured it would be God's will.

When she went back to the vascular specialist, he advised surgery, but mentioned that she could have a stroke on the operating table. Considering that my mother was in her eighties and didn't want surgery, the doctor agreed that it would probably be better for her not to have it. She lived several years afterwards without having a stroke that we were aware of.

No negative consequences resulted from the technologist showing my mother the results of her ultrasound report. There were, however, benefits. Here are some:

◆ She didn't have to go through the anxiety of wondering what her results were. It's often less stressful to know what the bad results are than to wonder if they are bad. Most people want to be told the results of tests as soon as they are known.

◆ She had time to formulate questions and consider the consequences of her blocked carotids before she saw the specialist. When people first hear bad news, they are often in a state of shock and unable to think rationally. It's usually better to make important decisions after a period of reflection.

◆ After the test, my mother was more motivated to watch her diet and take her cholesterol medication regularly. Her cholesterol did go down and the symptoms that prompted the rush visit to the vascular specialist gradually went away. In fact, in the last year and a half of her life, her doctor was able to take her off cholesterol drugs and still have her maintain a good cholesterol level.

◆ It was easier for the doctor to discuss the results and options for treatment because my mother already had prior knowledge of them.

◆ Seeing images of blocked arteries is a more effective motivating force than just hearing cholesterol statistics from your doctor. I think all people should be encouraged to see what their arteries look like during ultrasound exams and then compare them to an image of a normal artery.

◆ The ultrasound images of my mother's blocked carotids had a major impact on me. I immediately changed what I ate afterwards, and I watched my cholesterol more closely than I had before. Likewise, after I saw the images of my mother's spine and hip at her bone density center, I was more motivated to get tested and take preventive action.

Patients have to pay for their medical tests, consent to treatment, and suffer the consequences of whatever treatment is chosen. Therefore they should be allowed to communicate with technologists and see images of their body on x-rays and computer monitors if they wish to do so. Competent medical doctors don't just rely on written reports about images; they also look at the image. Patients should be able to do the same.

The protocol of having doctors tell patients the results of their tests was intended to benefit patients by assuring that they get information from the best qualified people. Fifty years ago, this practice worked because doctors had more time to spend with patients.

Nowadays, however, insurance companies are paying doctors less and less, so doctors have to increase their patient load in order to pay their expenses. HMO's (health maintenance organizations) are even instructing their doctors to reduce the amount of time they spend with patients. As a result, patients now spend less time with their physicians. Consequently, there is little time for doctors to discuss bone density results and give their patients preventive advice.

A solution to this dilemma is to let qualified technologists provide information to patients. There *is* time during the test for technologists to talk to patients and answer their questions. The problem is that they are often instructed to refer questions to the patient's doctor. If technologists were allowed to communicate with patients and show them the monitor, this would not only benefit the patient, it would also make the technologist's job more interesting and satisfying. They can be taught to present test results in a positive manner that still encourages patients to make changes that prevent bone loss. If the medical profession is committed to reducing osteoporosis, it should take advantage of every opportunity to educate patients about bone health.

Jewelry Appraisals and Bone Appraisals

During the period in which I formulated this book in my mind, I was writing a book entitled *Diamond Handbook: How to Look at Diamonds and Avoid Ripoffs.* It has a chapter on how to choose an appraiser and evaluate jewelry appraisals. I now realize that consumer tips on getting a jewelry appraisal can also apply to getting a bone appraisal—a bone density report.

In both cases, it's important that the report be thorough and contain pertinent details. An appraisal of a diamond ring, for example, must contain enough information to make sure that it will be replaced with a ring of equivalent quality if it is lost or stolen. American insurance companies seldom pay cash for jewelry. They usually just buy a replacement piece at wholesale.

A bone density report should provide enough detail to ensure that you get an accurate diagnosis. One that only has average spine and hip scores is not sufficient. A good density report of the hip and spine is usually at least four pages in length and includes:

◆ **The bone mineral densities (BMD) of various parts of the hip** including the femoral neck and trochanter, as well as the total hip.

◆ **The bone mineral density of each of the first four lumbar vertebrae** (L1, L2, L3, & L4). It should also include an average of all or some of these vertebrae. If any vertebrae show fractures or very noticeable arthritic changes, the doctor or radiologist may exclude them from the average spine BMD.

◆ **T-scores of the various sites on the hip and lumbar spine**. T-scores compare your bone densities with those of a large group of young adults.

◆ **Z-scores of the various sites on the hip and lumbar spine.** Z-scores compare your bone densities with those of a large group of people of your age and race.

◆ **Images of your lumbar vertebrae and hip(s).** They may resemble an X-ray with the most dense areas appearing white, or they may be a positive image with the most dense areas appearing black. If you get an original copy from the test center, the images will probably be clearer than if you get a photocopy of the report from your doctor In addition, if the report is in color, you'll be able to see the colors in the original.

◆ **A diagnosis**

◆ **A summary** which usually includes average T-scores

◆ **The model and manufacturer of the densitometer used**

◆ **The definitions used** to determine if you have normal bone mass, osteopenia or osteoporosis.

Bone density reports are not limited to the above information; they may also include other details such as your hip axis length, which can help doctors predict your risk of fracture.

The costs of bone density tests of the hip and spine typically range from $125–$180. Curiously, detailed reports that measure both hips may cost no more than reports that only provide general density data of the total spine and one hip. Similarly, bone density centers that allow patients to talk to their staff and get immediate feedback about the test results may charge no more than an imaging center that merely does the test. Therefore, it's to your advantage to ask testing places beforehand what's included in their reports, what services they offer, and whether they'll discuss the results with you.

Paying for Bone Density Testing

If you're 65 or older and you have specific osteoporosis risk factors, government health plans will usually pay for some form of bone density test. In the United States, Canada and some other countries, the cost of a DXA scan of the hip and spine is covered for seniors. In the US, the basic Medicare plan allows patients to select their own doctor and testing center. However, seniors with supplemental HMO Medicare policies are often limited in their choice of doctors and testing facilities. For more information, talk to your health care providers and see www.medicare.gov.

More and more insurance companies and government health plans are paying for density testing in people below the age of 65, depending on the circumstances. However, if your insurance plan has a high deductible that you haven't reached, you'll have to pay for the test even if it's covered by your insurance.

If your insurance won't pay for a DXA test and you think it would be helpful, don't hesitate to pay for it yourself. I've paid for mine; and some of my friends have, too, including my friend in France, whom I mentioned earlier. People who have money to pay for luxury items like sports cars, designer clothes or electronic goods should be able to pay for a bone density test. It all depends on your priorities.

When patients pay for a test, they tend to have higher expectations of the testing center. They want thorough documentation of their test results, and they want to be able to ask the staff relevant questions. As a consequence, they usually learn more from their tests than patients who are totally reimbursed.

Finding a Bone Density Center

Even though some bone density test centers are committed to educating their patients, it's not always easy to find them. If you'd like to be tested at an information-oriented center, consider doing some research in advance. For example, ask your friends and relatives about their experiences at density centers. Here are some types of questions you might wish to ask:

1. Were they able to talk to a doctor or technologist at the center?
2. Did anyone discuss the importance of exercise or suggest specific types of exercise they could do to help maintain bone mass?
3. Did anyone discuss diet or calcium-rich foods?
4. Did anyone discuss other nutrients besides calcium that are important for bone health?

5. Did anyone discuss the importance of posture or check their posture?

6. Did anyone mention osteoporosis risk factors or discuss how bone density can be affected by smoking, alcohol, caffeine, and certain types of medications such as corticosteroids and thyroid hormone?

7. Were they allowed to look at their spine and hip on the computer monitor?

8. Did anyone at the test center explain what a T-score is or how to interpret density test results?

9. Were there any books, booklets, magazines, brochures or fliers about bone health in the waiting room of the density center?

The answers don't all have to be positive, but in education-oriented testing centers, many of them will be.

Sometimes you can find DXA test centers on the Internet. For example, occasionally they may be listed under "osteoporosis center" in the Yahoo yellow pages.

Another way of finding bone density test centers is to ask your insurance company and to look through the list of doctors for your insurance plan. Osteoporosis specialists can sometimes be located under the specialty rheumatology, a branch of medicine that studies and treats disorders of the joints, bones and muscles. Rheumatologists that may have a densitometer sometimes list their office as an arthritis and osteoporosis medical center. This type of osteoporosis listing may only appear in an insurance company's written directory of physicians and not on their website.

There's no physician specialty yet dedicated to osteoporosis. However, there are doctors other than rheumatologists who may have a co-specialty of osteoporosis, including endocrinologists, gynecologists, orthopedists and internists. Some of these doctors may also do bone density testing.

One way to find these doctors is to check the National Osteoporosis Foundation website—www.nof.org. Click on "Find a Doctor," then select your state from the pull-down menu. Before you make an appointment, ask them to describe their bone density reports and find out how much of the practice is dedicated to osteoporosis. Make a good selection the first time because you'll have to do follow-up tests on the same densitometer if you want to accurately compare the results to the first test.

If you live outside the US, you can look for your national osteoporosis organization on the website of the International Osteoporosis Foundation:

http://www.osteofound.org/member_societies/societies.php

What to Do if There's No DXA Center in Your Area

In many small cities and rural areas, densitometers don't exist. Even in a major cosmopolitan city such as London, it can be a challenge finding a place that offers DXA tests of the spine and hip. In some countries, DXA spine and hip tests may be reserved for people who have had fractures or who have had heel or arm tests indicating very low bone densities.

If there are no DXA centers in your area and you're interested in getting tested, discuss this with your doctors and local hospitals. If they receive enough requests, they may decide to buy a densitometer. Meanwhile, consider getting tested out of town when you go on vacation or business trips or when you visit relatives.

You may also have to travel in order to find a doctor with specialized training in osteoporosis care. I know a jeweler with osteoporosis who traveled 600 miles (968 kilometers) to see an osteoporosis specialist because there were none in her hometown. She was glad she did.

Follow the guidelines in the preceding section for locating an out-of-town test center. If your doctor isn't familiar with DXA tests, try and go to a center with a physician who is able to recommend treatment if needed. Find out in advance if a doctor's order is required for the test. If you're paying for the test yourself and it's done in a doctor's office, you probably won't need a referral. However, imaging centers often require them.

Should a Doctor's Order Be Required for DXA Tests?

When insurance companies or government health plans pay for a DXA test, they may expect a physician to authorize the test and provide a referral slip; they don't want to spend money unless it's necessary. In this case, it's normal for DXA test centers to require a doctor's order. Otherwise, they may not be reimbursed.

However, when patients pay for the test themselves, it's difficult to understand why a doctor's order may be required, particularly when patients may be able to go to the same testing center and get a full body scan without a doctor's order. DXA tests are safe and use a lot less radiation than body scans.

There's no point in creating unnecessary paperwork for doctors when patients are paying for the test themselves. Doctors already have enough to do. Patients who pay shouldn't have to spend their time either getting referral slips. DXA tests provide valuable information, and it should be as easy as possible to get one.

Why You Should Study Your Density Reports Instead of Relying Solely on Your Doctors

I have competent doctors who focus just as much on prevention as on treatment. However, whether or not your doctor(s) emphasizes prevention, it's still helpful for you to study your own bone density reports. Below are some reasons why.

1. **You'll be able to alert other medical professionals about problem areas in your skeleton.** It's helpful for orthopedists, endocrinologists, physical therapists, chiropractors, yoga teachers, and trainers to know if you have osteoporosis or areas of low bone mass. The more you're able to tell professionals about your bones and your health, the better able they are to help you. However, they need specific information.

   For example, if a competent trainer or physical therapist knows the weakest areas of your spine or hip, they can show you which exercises will help you most. They can also show you the best form and placement for your body on resistance machines. Slight differences in the positioning of your feet and arms can change the target area of an exercise. If you have osteoporosis and they have specialized training in osteoporosis, these professionals can show you which exercises are safest for you. It helps if they know which areas of your body have very low bone density.

2. **Many doctors have never studied bone densitometry.** It's only been since the late 1980's that DXA bone density tests have been offered. In the last ten years, the advances in technology and introduction of new machines have occurred as fast as changes in computers. Consequently, general practitioners can't be expected to have a thorough knowledge of the latest developments in bone densitometry. It's a specialized field.

3. **Doctors are often overloaded with work and may not have much time to study your density reports.** The medical establishment typically has a triage system of tending to the most seriously ill patients first. Sometimes they are so busy examining the lab, MRI and x-ray reports of sick patients that they may not have much time to study the bone density reports of healthy people.

4. **You'll be more motivated to optimize your exercise routine and improve your diet** if you know you have potential problem areas in your spine or hip. You may also be more motivated to take measures to prevent falls. Seeing specific medical data on paper can be more motivating than hearing verbal summaries of your test results.

5. **Some doctors are more geared to treatment than to prevention.** They wait until a patient has osteoporosis to alert them of a problem. If you want to avoid osteoporosis, you have to take preventive measures before you get it. It's easier to prevent bone loss than to reverse it.

6. **Studying your reports can help you appreciate your doctors more.** Many people don't realize the amount of work doctors have in addition to seeing patients. When you see all the information there is on a bone density report and consider that doctors have piles of other reports to look at, along with insurance forms, prescriptions, and patient forms to fill out, you can better appreciate all that your doctor does. It will also help you put matters into perspective if a minor mistake occurs. Doctors are human beings with complicated jobs. They aren't infallible and you shouldn't expect them to be.

7. **Reading the details on your report can help you avoid becoming overconfident about your bone health.** On my last report, which was from an osteoporosis specialist, the assessment stated: "This patient is considered normal according to World Health Organization (WHO) criteria." However, in the same paragraph it also said, "The BMD measured at Femur Neck Right is 0.918 g/cm^2 with a T-score of -0.9. Bone density is up to 10% below young normal." In other words, the neck of my right hip (an area that's susceptible to fracture) was approaching low bone mass (osteopenia). This was despite the fact that my total right hip had a high T-score of +0.2.

   Seeing that comment at home made me realize that I should not get lazy about exercising my hips, especially since I was discontinuing drug therapy.

   Time restrictions during an office visit or bone density exam does not normally allow doctors to bring up these types of details. But even when they do mention them, you may not absorb and remember all the information. That's why it's helpful for you to study your reports.

How to Be a Savvy Patient

Savvy diamond buyers learn about diamonds before they buy them and do business with competent professionals. In addition, they get documentation verifying the quality, weight and authenticity of their diamonds.

Savvy patients who want to avoid osteoporosis should learn about the disease and ways to help prevent it. They should also have some knowledge about bone density exams before they're tested. This will better enable them to select a competent testing center that offers comprehensive reports.

Besides getting a copy of the bone density report, they should seek professional guidance in understanding their test results.

These days, it's fairly easy to find consumer information on buying a diamond, and many diamond buyers have a basic understanding of diamond color and clarity. Obtaining information about bone density testing is more difficult. Few patients who undergo DXA tests know the significance of their numerical results. Seldom do they receive a copy of their bone density report. This is despite the fact that a person's bone health should be much more important than the quality of their diamonds.

Reading this book is a good a way to start learning about osteoporosis prevention and bone density testing. However, it's also helpful to read health magazines, journals and other books. The appendix lists osteoporosis websites that can provide you with the latest findings about osteoporosis.

Previous sections provided tips on selecting bone density centers and evaluating the thoroughness of bone density reports. Below are some additional suggestions. If you'd like to have a DXA test:

◆ **Find out if your insurance company or government medical plan will pay for the test**. If they do, ask if a referral from your primary physician is necessary and if there are any other requirements for reimbursement. Even if your insurance or government plan pays for the bone density exam, a referral may not be needed if you are tested by a doctor. Find out beforehand.

◆ **Make sure the DXA center provides thorough reports** that include the densities and T-scores of the different areas of the hip and each of the lumbar vertebrae that are tested. The center may have a sample.

◆ **Schedule an appointment for a bone density test about a month or so before your annual physical**, if possible. That way you'll be able to get the report in time to discuss the results face-to-face with your regular doctor. Ask the center when the report will be ready. Some centers have the results ready the same day; others may take as long as a month to complete the report.

◆ **Review bone density terminology before the exam** so that your discussion with the doctor or technologist at the center will be more meaningful. For example, reread Chapter 4, "Basic Bone Terminology" and Chapters 13 and 14 on bone density reports and testing.

◆ **If the center doesn't offer to show you the images of your hip and spine on the monitor, ask to see them**. It's helpful to visually see your areas of high and low densities. One advantage of being tested by an osteoporosis specialist is that he or she can explain the images and give you information that you can't get from a book or from a general physician who hasn't studied bone densitometry.

◆ **Find out when the written report will be completed, and ask for two copies of it**—one for your regular doctor and one for yourself. The two reports should be originals from the densitometer so the images of your spine and hip are as clear as possible. Some test centers are able to give you the report at the time of the test.

◆ **Study the report before you see your general physician.** After you read it, you may have questions that were not answered at the test center. Take the report with you to your doctor so you can make notes on it.

◆ **Write down any questions you may have in the order of their importance.** Otherwise you may forget some of them, or you may waste valuable time on unimportant matters during your appointment. Time will be limited

◆ **If you have osteoporosis, get a referral to a physical therapist with a specialty in osteoporosis** from your regular doctor (or the osteoporosis specialist if you saw one). Proper exercise is one of the most important means of treatment and prevention, but some exercises are better and safer than others. You'll need to do more than walk. Physical therapy is typically covered by insurance and government medical plans, but check first to see if it's included in your plan. You or your doctor may have to do some research to find a therapist who has been trained to treat osteoporosis patients, but it's worth it to locate one.

In summary, to be a savvy patient, you should:

◆ Learn about osteoporosis and bone density tests before you're tested and see your doctor.

◆ Get tested at a competent, information-oriented center, who will answer your questions.

◆ Verify in advance that you will receive a detailed bone density report.

◆ Write down the most important questions you may have about your test results and treatment options before you see your doctor.

16

Pros & Cons of Giving Patients their Medical Reports

In the United States, doctors and medical institutions are required by law to give patients copies of their medical records. However, patients usually have to request the copies. In France, on the other hand, patients typically get copies of their test results without having to ask.

In the fall of 2003, I visited France. While I was there, I asked a friend about the results of her bone density test. She showed me the copy of the five-page report the testing center had given her a half hour after she was tested. The center also sent a copy to her doctor who would have recommended treatment if it had been necessary.

My friend was surprised when I told her that it's not customary for US labs and testing centers to give patients copies of their reports. She then showed me all of the lab results, mammograms, and x-rays that had been given to her since she was 21. Later she sent me an article entitled, "How to Read your Lab Results." It was from the November 2003 issue of Cosmopolitan Magazine (French edition, p 62). It advised readers to save all their lab reports as a basis of comparison.

Many doctors in America tend to notify patients of their test results only when there's a problem. Even if the news is bad, some doctors don't provide specific verbal data. They may just say, for example, "your cholesterol is high."

The American practice of not offering information to patients has not helped them improve their health. Americans have a higher incidence of heart disease and obesity, and they take more pills than people in France.

Why Keeping Copies of Your Test Results Comes in Handy

A casual comment by a physician in Hong Kong prompted me to start asking my doctors for copies of my lab reports. I went to him because of a high fever and chest congestion. While the doctor was looking at the results of my blood tests, he said, "If I knew what your blood work was when you were well, it would be easier to determine how sick you are."

That happened in 1984. Ever since, I've asked my doctors for written copies of my lab tests so that I'd be able to provide any physician with details of my medical history. I've never had a problem obtaining the copies. I was an international tour director then, and I knew that if I fell ill while on tour, it would be difficult to get information quickly from a doctor in the United States.

Even though I never again needed to see a doctor while traveling abroad, copies of my test results have come in handy because:

◆ The doctor I had in the mid 1980's moved out of town; nevertheless I have my records for that period of time, which I can still use for comparison purposes.

◆ My next doctor had his license suspended. Providing another doctor with my records was no problem because I had copies of them.

◆ Having the copies of the test results has allowed me to compare them and see how my diet and activities have affected them over the years.

◆ My doctors normally haven't had to spend time and money sending my records to insurance companies or other physicians. I provided the copies when needed.

Doctors' Concerns about Giving Patients their Medical Reports

Some US doctors automatically give patients copies of their lab and bone density tests. Most do not, however, unless the patient asks for the copies. Some of the concerns these doctors have are:

1. The reports may be too difficult for a patient to understand.

2. Patients may misinterpret the results.

3. The test results may make the patients worry and overreact.

4. Patients may use the results for a lawsuit.

The saying "A little knowledge is a dangerous thing" sums up the concerns of these doctors.

I firmly believe that patients should examine their medical reports, so I shall address each of the above concerns.

1. **The reports may be too difficult for a patient to understand:** This is true in some cases, but patients can always skip over what they don't understand. The more they examine their reports, the easier it is to interpret them, especially since the normal and out-of-range results are usually indicated. If asked, most doctors would be willing to explain the most important points. In fact, good doctors consider this their job.

2. **Patients may misinterpret the results.** This is also true. However, misinterpretations can be corrected, and you can ask your doctor and other professionals to help you interpret the results.

3. **The test results may make the patients worry and overreact.** I agree. I overreacted to the results of my bone density report, but that didn't hurt me. Instead it motivated me to do research on osteoporosis and make constructive changes that I otherwise wouldn't have made. For example, I never would have signed up for strength training lessons had I not seen my written results. The training helped reverse the downward trend of my bone density. It also increased my muscle strength and helped improve my balance.

   Many people are like me. They need to get upset in order to take action that will benefit them. Protecting patients from worry by not giving them their test results can do more harm than good. It's better for people to get scared while in good health than to end up in a hospital and then learn they must change their habits.

4. **Patients may use the results for a lawsuit**. That's possible, but if people want to sue, they'll request their medical reports anyway. I believe that patients who take responsibility for their health and study their test results are more likely to blame themselves for their health problems than their doctors. Proactive patients are also more likely to recognize symptoms of disease and get proper care before a problem becomes serious. In addition, they may notice errors on reports and alert their doctor. This can help the doctor avoid improper treatment and a lawsuit.

   Joel Figatner, MD, an urgent-care and former family-practice physician, agrees. He says that in the U.S., it's not a matter of if a doctor will be sued, but when. Dr. Figatner believes that a key to minimizing lawsuits is to establish good rapport with patients, and that involves helping them interpret their medical reports. Informed patients are more likely to feel genuine rapport with him and are less likely to sue if the outcome does not go as anticipated.

   The cost of lawsuits makes malpractice insurance rates rise, which in turn can lead to higher hospital and medical costs. A decrease in lawsuits would help to lower the startling rate of increase for health insurance premiums for American consumers. The medical profession could help lower the number of lawsuits if it would encourage patients to examine their medical reports and take more responsibility for their health.

Doctors Who Show Patients Their Medical Reports

More and more doctors are voluntarily giving patients copies of their test results. They realize that when patients are involved with their health care, they are more likely to follow their doctor's advice. For example, I have stopped eating most junk food because I have seen over the years how it has affected my test results and the health of my family. I used to eat a large package of cookies or chips in a day, but those days are over, even though I have no weight problems.

Dr. Figatner routinely gave patients in his family practice copies of their test results because providing them with written documentation:

◆ Allowed patients to keep a file of their medical records at home

◆ Encouraged patients to take responsibility for their wellness

◆ Allowed patients to track their progress over the years

◆ Let patients research topics and questions on the Internet

◆ Prevented delays and omissions in transferring medical records to a new doctor when the patients moved. Sometimes patients' files are as thick as a book. It's time consuming for a physician to go through all the records and determine which reports are the most relevant for the next doctor. Reports from previous doctors are not necessarily recopied. If a patient wants a new physician to have a complete file of his or her health, it's best for the patient to provide a copy of that file to the new doctor.

As an urgent-care physician, Dr. Figatner now routinely gives copies of medical reports to patients who transfer to a higher level of care or who require timely follow-up so that they'll have records for the other doctor(s).

Dr. Figatner also shows his patients their x-rays because he finds one picture is worth 10,000 words. It's easier to explain with pictures than with medical terminology. Most people, for example, don't know the names of the bones. But if they see a bone on film, they can understand what it is. In addition, the film allows the whole family to see the results and be involved in the patient's care.

Dr. Figatner has observed that patients above 60 years of age often expect their doctor to function as an all-knowing giver, whereas the patient is the unquestioning receiver. Younger patients in their 40's and below tend to have different expectations of their doctor: Their attitude says "treat me as a partner in my health care. Give me options and help me interpret my tests. But let me participate in the medical decisions."

Another doctor, Marie Savard, MD, wrote a book telling patients why they should collect copies of all of their medical records—*How to Save*

Your Own Life. She states that in today's rapidly changing HMO (Health Maintenance Organization) culture, the doctor you see at today's visit may be a totally different doctor next time. On page xiii of her book, Savard brings up the case of the insolvent HIP health Plan of New Jersey. On the last day of operation, workers had to deal with crowds of panicky patients trying to obtain their own records for the first time. She also mentions that if you don't collect your records, they can lawfully be destroyed after two to seven years, by the people and facilities that own them (p. 27). Information on Savard's books can be found at www.drsavard.com.

While writing this book, I met a nurse who was in charge of computerizing the charts of a medical group of doctors in the northwestern United States. She told me that the medical professionals in the group could now easily show patients their charts on the computer screen. By doing so, they have seen a major increase in patients' adherence to doctors' recommendations. Patients who had previously ignored their doctor's advice to get follow-up tests and take medications now did what their doctor suggested after seeing their test results. And patients were more comfortable with the use of computers when they knew their doctors were not hiding anything from them.

Patient compliance was greatest when they were shown graphs of their test results over the years along with the latest results. I can relate to this. When I saw my bone density results in the summer of 2003, I was more concerned about the 7.3 per cent decrease in my hip density than about the low bone mass (osteopenic) level of my spine, which had gone down 2.9 per cent. My spine scores prompted my density center and doctor to recommend drug therapy. But the downward trend of my hip density is what spurred me most to take other preventive action too. That's why it's important for patients to have records of past results.

I need to visually see things on paper or on a computer screen in order to understand them. I can't assimilate material by just hearing a doctor briefly explain it. Even when I do see my results on paper, I need to reread them several times. Humans remember information better when it is repeated and when it is both seen and heard. Doctors who realize this go beyond verbal advice. They also show patients their medical information, be it on paper, on a computer screen or in the form of x-rays.

The maxim "a little knowledge is a dangerous thing" should not be used as an excuse to avoid offering patients copies of their medical results. It should instead encourage doctors to provide patients with more knowledge. A patient's medical record is not only one of the best sources of information; it's also one of the best motivational tools available.

17

Hip and Spine Density Tests: A Case Study

I've had more DXA bone density exams than the average person because I was curious about the effects of alendronate (Fosamax®) and various types of exercise on my bones, particularly during the period around menopause. Some research studies measure bone density every six months, and ever since being diagnosed with low bone mass, I've had tests done almost as frequently. If density tests are done this often outside of a formal research study, the patient has to pay for them, which is appropriate.

My Bone Density Exams

My first three DXA tests were done at an imaging center, which I will call Test Center A. They provided good, detailed reports, but they only did the test. They did not offer preventive advice, discuss the test results or show me the computer images of my spine and hip. When I scheduled my third exam, I asked if I'd be able to pose questions about my previous density report. The center's policy is to refer questions about test results to the patient's doctor. However, it would be at least six months before I saw my doctor for a physical. I wanted my questions answered before then. In addition, my doctor did not have direct access to the images and data of my test and wouldn't be able to show them to me on the computer screen.

I decided then that I'd prefer to get future tests done some place where I could discuss the test results with the staff. As a result, I switched to my mother's testing center, the one who first advised me to get a DXA bone density test of my spine and hip. In this book, I refer to it as Test Center B.

I knew that I couldn't accurately compare my past or future test results with those of another testing center. Consequently, I got two sets of tests done within a period of nine days—one at Test Center A to compare previous results and one at Test Center B to start a new baseline.

Test Center B offered preventive advice, discussed my preliminary results, showed me the images on the monitor, answered my questions about previous tests, and gave me a written sheet explaining osteoporosis risk factors and T-scores. In addition, they measured both hips instead of just one. There were no additional charges for these services. The computer results had to be analyzed by a radiologist, who gave summaries and recommendations on a report, which I received later.

While doing research for this book, I learned that some osteoporosis specialists also give bone density exams. They offer the same services as Test Center B, but they're able to give a definitive diagnosis at the time of the exam and answer any questions you have about it. The cost of the test can be the same as what one would pay at an imaging center, about $125 to $180. Insurance companies typically establish a maximum amount that they will pay for bone density testing. Normally this maximum applies whether or not the center has a professional qualified to discuss the results. After I learned the benefits of osteoporosis specialists, I decided to go to one. Later in this chapter, I briefly discuss my visit there (see page 152).

Four-year Study of the Changes in My Bone Densities

Most bone-density studies are planned carefully in advance. This one wasn't. I didn't start doing research on osteoporosis until the summer of 2003—2½ years after my first bone density test at Test Center A. At that time, I didn't know there were two types of bone gain and loss—systemic and localized. I only knew that there was a wide variation in the T-scores and bone densities throughout my hip and lumbar spine. I didn't know why.

After doing research and comparing my test results at 6–9-month intervals, I learned that exercise has a localized effect on my bones. When examining four years of test results, I could see a direct correlation between the densities of my various skeletal areas and the amount and type of exercise they receive. I could also see an overall systemic loss of bone that occurred just prior to menopause before taking alendronate (Fosamax).

Since three of my tests were done at Test Center A and three were done at Test Center B, I can't use the T-scores or BMD (bone mineral density) figures as an accurate means of comparison for the four-year period. Therefore, I've decided to compare the percentage decreases and increases of my bone densities for the pairs of tests done on the same densitometer. Even though this method has its limitations, it can indicate general trends in my bone densities. First I'll review spine and hip terminology with two photos.

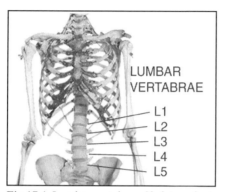

Fig 17.1 Lumbar vertebrae. *Skeleton photo courtesy of www.skullsunlimited.com.*

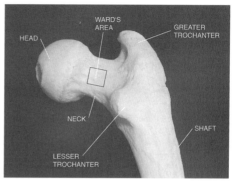

Fig. 17.2 Femoral hip. *Photo by Ed Newton.*

Percentage changes in my spine densities during four years*

AP Spine	#1 (age 52–55) Winter 2001– Summer 2003 2½-year period	#2 (age 55) Summer 2003 – Winter 2004 7 months	#3 (age 55–56) Winter 2004 – Fall 2004 9 months	#4 (age 56–57) Fall 2004 – Spring 2005 6 months
Test Center	Center A	Center A	Center B	Center B
L1 BMD%	+0.59%	+1.98%	-4.54%	+4.1%
L2 BMD%	-9.03%	+10.65%	-1.07%	+3.44%
L3 BMD%	-2.89%	-5.61%	+0.34%	+1.69%
L2–L3 BMD%**	-2.94%	+1.8%	-0.35%	+2.62%
L1–L3 BMD%	—	—	-1.73%	+3.06%

*   The percentage changes were calculated from the bone mineral densities (BMD's) on my reports, which are listed later in the chapter. The formula for determining the percentage change in BMD is:
   (BMD of current test - BMD of previous test) ÷ BMD of previous test

** Test Center A used L2–L3 to establish their spine score. The ancillary results of Test Center B listed the T-scores of various combinations of lumbar vertebrae.

Trends in the spine densities during the four periods:

#1 A decrease in the density of my lumbar spine (L2–L3)
#2 An increase in the overall density of my lumbar spine
#3 A decrease in the density of the lumbar spine
#4 An increase in bone density throughout the lumbar spine

Percentage changes in my left hip densities during four years

Left Hip	#1 Winter 2001 – Summer 2003 2½-year period	#2 Summer 2003 – Winter 2004 7 months	#3 Winter 2004 – Fall 2004 9 months	#4 Fall 2004 – Spring 2005 6 months
Test Center	Center A	Center A	Center B	Center B
neck BMD %	-7.78%	-0.78%	+0.8%	+5.87%
trochanter BMD%	-10.42%	+5.2%	+2.81%	+2.6%
shaft BMD%	-2.5%	+1.28%	+0.08%	+3.02%
total hip BMD%	-7.28%	+3.41%	+0.92%	+2.13%

Trends in the hip densities during the four periods:

#1 A significant decrease in the densities of my hip

#2 A significant increase of my total hip and trochanter

#3 A non-significant increase in the densities of my hip

#4 Greater increases in the densities of the hip than in period #3

#1– #4 The bone density of the shaft of my leg remained relatively stable.

Overall trend during the four periods

During the first period, my bone density went down, especially in the hip. After that it tended to go up, particularly during the fourth period. One exception was in period #3 when the spine density went down.

Bone loss and gain is not accidental. To determine what causes it in my body, I must analyze the factors that remain consistent and those that change. The next section discusses the consistencies.

Factors that remained the same throughout all four periods:

◆ My combined intake of calcium from food and supplements was at least 1200 mg per day

◆ My intake of vitamin D was over 400 IU (international units) per day and I was in a climate with lots of sunshine.

◆ The brand and type of calcium supplement remained the same— Citracal® Plus (calcium citrate) with magnesium oxide, vitamin D and other bone nutrients.

◆ I did at least 12 hours of weight-bearing exercise per week, which included walking, running and dancing.

◆ I ate a well-balanced diet which included whole grains, dairy products, seafood, poultry, meat, eggs, beans, nuts, and at least eight servings of fruits and vegetables each day.

◆ I had no health problems.

Despite these consistencies, there was a significant variation in my bone densities from one period to another. Let's look at some differences.

Factors that changed during the four periods

◆ During the first two periods, I was approaching menopause, which I reached by the third period. As women enter menopause, their estrogen levels plunge, causing them to lose the bone-preserving benefits of estrogen. Losing bone at this time is normal. What is not usual is to have gains in bone density during the first year following menopause, particularly during a period of only six-months.

◆ During the last three periods, I took a 70-mg alendronate (Fosamax) pill once a week. Nevertheless, in the third period, my spine bone density went down, even though I was on alendronate. It probably would have gone down more without the alendronate.

◆ During the last three periods, I added soy products to my diet (mainly tofu) because they contain plant estrogens, which may help offset the decline in estrogen which occurs around menopause. Soy products did not prevent bone loss in my spine during the third period.

◆ During most of the second period, I attended two extra yoga classes per week. I didn't attend any after the second period, but in the third period, I started to do exercises for the hip. During Period 4, the period of greatest bone gain, I weight trained and did hip exercises.

◆ At the beginning of Period 3, I strained some back muscles for the second time doing yoga. As a result I stopped attending yoga classes and decreased the amount of lifting in my everyday activities. Instead I did posture and back exercises such as shoulder pullbacks and upper body resistance exercises, which involved pressing hard against a large ball and pulling on two ends of a towel. Despite these back exercises, lots of walking, and my weekly alendronate pill, the density of my spine went down during the third period. Nevertheless, the back exercises did help improve my posture. My results suggest that my spine also requires weight training, which can challenge it by placing gradually increasing loads on the vertebrae.

◆ After seeing on my winter 2004 report that my right hip had better bone density than my left, I noticed that I tended to rest on my right hip more often than on my left when I stood. I tried to even out my weight more when I walked, and I started shifting my weight more to my left leg when I was standing. Perhaps the weight shift was responsible for decreasing the difference in densities between my right and left hips.

My overall conclusions

It appears that Fosamax was effective at stopping my bone loss. However, I needed to do site-specific exercise to show bone gains. The greatest gains occurred when I was doing weight-training. General hip exercises and yoga also appear to have been helpful at increasing bone density in my hip.

My test results indicate that I was able to reverse the declining densities of my hip and spine with strength training and drug therapy. However, I don't know if I can do that with strength training alone. After I saw that my results were in the normal range in the spring of 2005, I decreased the amount of alendronate I was taking to one pill every two weeks at first and then to one every four weeks until my prescription ran out. After my next test, I'll know more about the effect of drug therapy and strength training on my bones.

Some sources state that it's pointless to get tested at intervals of less than a year because bone density changes too slowly to be noticeable at such intervals. During two different intervals of less than seven months each, I had bone gains of more than 3%, which is considered statistically significant. However, if I had only taken drugs, there may not have been any change; or worse yet, my densities may have declined. Bones need stimulation from activity and exercise in order to grow and be strong. I don't know of any clinical trials that have that have studied the effects of drugs in combination with exercise targeted to skeletal areas of low density.

My Bone Density Data

When people make claims about reversals in bone density, they should be able to back them up. This section provides detailed data from my reports at Test Centers A and B. Since the exams involved two different densitometers, you'll be able to see how bone density reports can vary depending on the densitometer. This doesn't mean that bone density tests aren't valid and useful; it simply means that you must consider the densitometer used when interpreting the results. Ideally, repeat tests should be done at the *same* test center and on the *same* machine as before (See *Journal of Clinical Densitometry*, vol. 7, no. 1, 2004). Even though there were significant differences in the data on the reports of each testing center, they both diagnosed me with osteopenia and suggested drug therapy, except in spring 2005, when I was diagnosed as normal.

Since both Centers A and B provided comprehensive reports supported by lots of data, I'm able to provide a thorough bone density study of my spine and hip in this section. For some people, the tables of data may be too thorough. They can be easily skipped, but some of the comments might be helpful. Medical professionals may be interested in the technical information; and people who want to understand their own bone density reports may also find some of the data useful. Therefore, it has been included in this section.

The tables on the following pages illustrate three principal points:

1. **The T-scores and BMD's (bone mineral densities) of individual sites should be considered** along with averaged BMD's and broad-area sites. My total hip T-scores are similar to those of a healthy thirty-year-old, but my femoral neck T-scores have sometimes been in the osteopenia (low bone mass) range, which is important for me to know.

   Even though the T-scores of my right and left hips aren't significantly different, those of some people are. It's better to look at the T-scores of each hip than to average their BMD's and just use the corresponding average T-scores for diagnosis; the hip with the lowest densities has the highest fracture risk.

2. **Significant differences may exist between the results of tests done on different densitometers**. However, new machines are getting more precise and may show little difference in their results.

3. **The general lumbar spine score should be determined on an individualized basis, not by a default computer setting**. Some densitometers measure L2–L4, the second to fourth lumbar vertebrae on their default setting. Newer machines tend to measure L1–L4. The divergent T-scores of my lumbar vertebrae are an example of why sometimes certain vertebrae should be excluded from the lumbar spine score so as to avoid falsely elevated scores. In my case, it's best to exclude L4.

As I explained in Chapter 13, **T-scores** tell how far your bone density deviates from that of a young adult. **Z-scores** compare your bone density to that of other people of the same age. The **BMD** value indicates the density of a specified area of your skeleton, without any reference to another person. The T-score is used for diagnosing osteoporosis and osteopenia, whereas the BMD is used for determining the percentage of your bone loss or gain between tests. Low Z-scores can prompt doctors to check if factors other than aging or menopause are causing bone loss.

T-scores and BMD* of my lumbar (lower) spine

(See Chapter 4 for an explanation of spine terminology and L1, L2, L3 & L4.)

	Winter 2001	Summer 2003	Winter 2004	Winter** 2004	Fall 2004	Spring 2005
Test Center	Center A	Center A	Center A	Center B	Center B	Center B
L1 T-score	-2.3	-2.3	-2.1	-1.4	-1.8	-1.4
L1 BMD	0.854	0.859	0.876	0.970	0.926	0.964
L2 T-score	-1.1	-1.9	-1.1	-0.8	-0.9	-0.5
L2 BMD	1.063	0.967	1.07	1.118	1.106	1.144
L3 T-score	-0.8	-0.5	-1.0	-0.3	-0.3	-0.1
L3 BMD	1.108	1.14	1.076	1.176	1.180	1.200
L4 T-score	+1.7	+1.5	+3.7	+1.3	+1.1	+1.4
L4 BMD	1.4	1.386	1.642	1.391	1.363	1.393
L2–L3***	-1.0	-1.2	-1.1	-0.5	-0.6	-0.3
L2–L3 BMD	1.086	1.054	1.073	1.148	1.144	1.174
L1–L3	—	—	—	-0.7	-0.8	-0.6
L1–L3 BMD				1.097	1.078	1.111
L1–L4	—	—	—	-0.1	-0.2	0
L1–L4 BMD				1.188	1.165	1.196

* BMD = bone mineral density

** This Test Center B test was done nine days apart from the Winter 2004 Center A test. There can be a significant difference in the scores depending on the densitometer used.

*** Test Center A only listed one general spine T-score on their reports—that of L2–L3.

T-score scale: Normal — above -1:
Low bone mass (osteopenia) — Between -1.0 and -2.5:
Osteoporosis — -2.5 and below

Comments:

◆ The spine score varies depending on the vertebral group selected. Since my 4th lumbar vertebra (L4) has an unusually high density, it's best not to use it for my spine score. Otherwise, the spine density will be falsely elevated.

◆ The way T-scores are determined can vary from one test center to another.

T-scores and BMD of my left femoral hip*

(See Chapter 4 for an explanation of the hip terminology used below)

	Winter 2001	Summer 2003	Winter 2004	Winter 2004**	Fall 2004	Spring 2005
Test Center	Center A	Center A	Center A	Center B	Center B	Center B
neck T-score	0	-0.7	-0.7	-1.3	-1.1	-0.7
neck BMD	0.977	0.901	0.894	0.878	0.885	0.937
trochanter T	+0.2	-0.5	-0.2	-.0	-0.7	-0.5
troch BMD	0.816	0.731	0.769	0.747	0.768	0.788
Wards*** T	-1.1	-1.8	-1.9	-1.6	-1.5	-1.2
Wards BMD	0.761	0.672	0.663	0.702	0.720	0.759
shaft BMD	1.281	1.249	1.265	1.240	1.239	1.265
total hip T	+0.4	-0.3	0	-0.3	-0.2	0
total hip BMD	1.044	0.968	1.001	0.976	0.985	1.006

* Only one hip was tested at Test Center A. Both were done at Center B.

** This Center B test was done nine days apart from the Winter 2004 Center A test. There can be a significant difference in the scores depending on the densitometer used.

*** The data for the Wards area is not normally used to diagnose osteoporosis. The T-scores of the trochanter, femoral neck and total hip are more important.

T-score scale: Normal — above -1.0

Low bone mass (osteopenia) — between -1.0 and -2.5

Osteoporosis — -2.5 and below

Comments:

◆ Even though the bone density of the left femoral neck was good in the winter of 2001, it was in the beginning stages of osteopenia in the winter and fall of 2004. This suggested that I needed to do site-specific exercises for the hip in order to help maintain bone mass there. I was already taking alendronate.

◆ My total hip scores are almost as good as those of a young adult, based on my T-scores. They could give me a false sense of security if I didn't consider the individual skeletal sites of the hip. Pay attention to the T-scores of the trochanter and femoral hip because these areas are where the hip is most likely to fracture.

T-scores and age-matched Z-scores of my lumbar (lower) spine

(See Chapter 4 for explanation of T-scores and Z-scores)

	Winter 2001	Summer 2003	Winter 2004	Winter 2004	Fall 2004	Spring 2005
Test Center	Center A	Center A	Center A	Center B	Center B	Center B
L1 T-score	-2.3	-2.3	-2.1	-1.4	-1.8	-1.4
L1 Z-score	-1.5	-1.2	-1.1	-0.4	-0.7	-0.3
L2 T-score	-1.1	-1.9	-1.1	-0.8	-0.9	-0.5
L2 Z-score	-0.4	-0.9	0	+0.2	+0.2	+0.6
L3 T-score	-0.8	-0.5	-1	-0.3	-0.3	-0.1
L3 Z-score	0	+0.5	0	+0.7	+0.7	+1.0
L4 T-score	+1.7	+1.5	+3.7	+1.3	+1.1	+1.4
L4 Z-score	+2.4	+2.6	+4.7	+2.3	+2.1	+2.5
L2–L3 T	-1.0	-1.2	-1.1	-0.5	-0.6	-0.3
L2–L3 Z	-0.2	-0.2	0	+0.5	+0.5	+0.8
L1–L3 T	—	—	—	-0.7	-0.8	-0.6
L1–L3 Z	—	—	—	+0.3	+0.2	+0.5
L1–L4 T	—	—	—	-0.1	-0.2	0
L1–L4 Z	—	—	—	+0.9	+0.8	+1.1

T-score scale: Above -1.0 — Normal compared to the average young adult
-1.0 to -2.5 — Low bone mass (osteopenia)
-2.5 and below — Osteoporosis

Z-score scale: 0   — Average value for people of the same age and gender
-1.0 — One standard deviation below average age-matched value
-2.0 — Two standard deviations below average age-matched value. A Z-score below this should prompt a thorough evaluation for causes of bone loss other than age and estrogen deficiency so the problem can be corrected (p 16 of *Bone Densitometry for Technologists* by Sydney Bonnick, MD, FACP and Lori Ann Lewis, MRT, CDT).

Comments:

◆ Overall the Z-scores of my lumbar spine are higher than those of other women my age, except for those of L1.

T-scores and Z-scores of my left femoral hip

	Winter 2001	Summer 2003	Winter 2004	Winter 2004*	Fall 2004	Spring 2005
Test Center	Center A	Center A	Center A	Center B	Center B	Center B
femoral neck T-score	0	-0.7	-0.7	-1.3	-1.1	-0.7
neck Z-score	+0.7	+0.3	+0.2	0	0	+0.5
trochanter T	+0.2	-0.5	-0.2	-1	-0.7	-0.5
troch Z-score	+0.6	-0.1	+0.3	0	+0.2	+0.4
Wards T-score	-1.1	-1.8	-1.9	-1.6	-1.5	-1.4
Wards Z-score	-0.1	-0.5	-0.6	-0.2	0	+0.1
total hip T	+0.4	-0.3	0	-0.3	-0.2	0
total hip Z	+0.9	+0.5	+0.7	+0.5	+0.2	+0.9

*   This Center B test was done nine days apart from the Winter 2004 Center A test. There can be a significant difference in the scores depending on the densitometer used.

T-score scale: Above -1.0 — Normal compared to the average young adult
-1.0 to -2.5 — Low bone mass (osteopenia)
-2.5 and below — Osteoporosis

Z-score scale: 0   — Average value for people of the same age and gender
-1.0 — One standard deviation below average age-matched value
-2.0 — Two standard deviations below average age-matched value. A Z-score below this should prompt a thorough evaluation for causes of bone loss other than age and estrogen deficiency so the problem can be corrected (p 16 of *Bone Densitometry for Technologists* by Sydney Bonnick, MD, FACP and Lori Ann Lewis, MRT, CDT).

Comments:

◆ With the exception of the density of the Ward's area, which is not normally used for diagnosis, the densities of my hip areas are the same or above that of the average woman my age.

◆ The downward trend of my hip densities from 2001–2003 was reversed between 2004–2005, suggesting that my preventive measures against osteoporosis were working.

T-Scores & BMD done nine days apart on different densitometers

Test Center	Winter 2004	Winter 2004
	Center A	Center B
L1 T-score	-2.1	-1.4
L1 BMD	0.876	0.970
L2 T-score	-1.1	-0.8
L2 BMD	1.070	1.118
L3 T-score	-1.0	-0.3
L3 BMD	1.076	1.176
L4 T-score	+3.7	+1.3
L4 BMD	1.642	1.391
L2–L3	-1.1	-0.5
L2–L3 BMD	1.073	1.148

Comments:

◆ The T-scores of my vertebrae were significantly higher at Center B, except for L4.

◆ Note how divergent the T-scores of individual vertebrae can be. Including all of them in the spine measurement can sometimes lead to falsely elevated spine T-scores. In my case, it's best to exclude L4 from the lumbar spine T-score.

Test Center	Winter 2004	Winter 2004
	Center A	Center B
femoral neck T-score	-0.7	-1.3
femoral neck BMD	0.894	0.878
trochanter T-score	-0.2	-1.0
trochanter BMD	0.769	0.747
shaft BMD	1.265	1.240
total hip T-score	0	-0.3
total BMD	1.001	0.976

◆ Curiously, the T-scores of my hip areas were higher at Center A, the opposite of my spine results.

◆ Even though the total-hip T-scores were almost as good as those of a young adult on both densitometers, the trochanter and femoral neck, were in the beginning stages of osteopenia on Center B's machine.

Moral: The densitometer used is an important consideration when comparing DXA results. For accurate comparison, follow-up tests should be done on the same densitometer.

The following year, I was tested by an osteoporosis specialist on a third densitometer two months after my Spring 2005 test. It was the same brand as the one at Test Center B, but a different model. The T-scores of the total left hip, left trochanter, right femoral neck, and spine (L1-L3) were identical to those of the Spring 2005 test. Otherwise, the average T-score difference of the sites used for diagnosis was just -0.1. Densitometers are becoming more and more precise.

Simplified Tables of my Results at Test Center B

Lumbar spine T-scores

Lumbar spine	Winter 2004	Fall 2004 9 months later	Spring 2005 6 months later
L1 T-score	-1.4	-1.8	-1.4
L2 T-score	-0.8	-0.9	-0.5
L3 T-score	-0.3	-0.3	-0.1
L1–L3 T-score	-0.7	-0.8	-0.6

Left femoral hip T-scores

Left hip	Winter 2004	Fall 2004 9 months later	Spring 2005 6 months later
femoral neck T-score	-1.3	-1.1	-0.7
trochanter T-score	-1.0	-0.7	-0.5
total hip T-score	-0.3	-0.2	0.0

Right femoral hip T-scores

Right hip	Winter 2004	Fall 2004 9 months later	Spring 2005 6 months later
femoral neck T-score	-0.7	-1.0	-0.9
trochanter T-score	-0.6	-0.4	-0.3
total hip T-score	+0.1	+0.1	+0.3

T-score scale

above -1.0	Normal
between -1.0 and -2.5	Low bone mass (osteopenia)
-2.5 and below	Osteoporosis

Follow-up Visit with an Osteoporosis Specialist

After I received my spring 2005 bone density report, I decided to make an appointment to discuss the results with an osteoporosis specialist (Test Center C). He had a new densitometer, which was the same brand but a different model than the one I'd been tested on two months earlier. I was curious to see if my results would also be normal on his machine. In addition, I wanted to establish a baseline at a testing place more conveniently located than Test Center B, which was four hours from my home. After showing him the results of my two previous tests, I was retested on his densitometer.

I was surprised at how similar the results were to those on the previous machine. The T-scores of the total left hip, left trochanter, right femoral neck, and spine (L1-L3) were identical. There was only a -0.1 deviation in the other three diagnostic areas, an acceptable margin of error and/or a possible change in two months. See table below:

T-scores two months apart in 2005

	Center B	Center C
Spine L1–L3	-0.6	-0.6
Trochanter left	-0.5	-0.5
Trochanter right	-0.3	-0.4
Neck left	-0.7	-0.8
Neck right	-0.9	-0.9
Total hip left	0	0
Total hip right	+0.3	+0.2

Given the normal results, the doctor said I could discontinue the alendronate (Fosamax) that I had been taking. However, since I had so many risk factors, he also presented the option of taking a preventive dose of half the amount of the drug. During the previous two months, I had already cut back to taking alendronate only once every two weeks instead of once a week. I decided to finish the remaining pills by taking them once a month and then discontinue the drug. This will allow me to compare the effects of strength training with and without alendronate.

The doctor recommended that I be retested in a year to check if my density is still stabilized without the alendronate. During just one visit to an osteoporosis specialist I had a bone density exam, and I received a diagnosis, treatment recommendations, preventive tips, and answers to my questions. I was 100% satisfied with the experience.

Don't Be Duped by Testimonials

When you see ads for bone-boosting products, they frequently include testimonials about increases in bone density such as:

Ad 1. "I've taken X product for two months and my doctor just told me that my bone density jumped from -2.5 to -1.9. I was so excited. I can already feel my bones getting stronger."

Ad 2. "My doctor said 'Wow!' when he saw my spine density had increased 21% from where it was a year ago. I owe this success to miracle product X."

Before believing such claims, find out:

◆ **What does the ad mean by "bone density?"** Is the testimonial referring to the density of the finger, heel, total hip and/or the lumbar spine? The preceding tables of my test results show how a person can have a wide range of bone densities, from low to high. Tests of a single skeletal site can give misleading results. When I state in this book that my bone density went up after I started strength training, that means it increased throughout the hip and lumbar spine.

◆ **Did the patient verify that the same densitometer was used for the comparison tests?** Major differences in bone densities can occur when a patient is measured on different densitometers.

◆ **What does the ad mean by "spine density?"** Depending on which vertebrae you include in the spine measurement, you can get very different results. Bone density centers differ in the way they determine the T-scores of the spine. When testimonials claim abnormally high increases such as 21% within a year in the spine or hip, be suspicious. An error may have occurred, the densitometer may have changed, the way of determining the spine T-scores may have been different, or the patient may have had vertebral fractures or arthritic changes, which could have led to falsely elevated T-scores.

◆ **What other factors may have contributed to the increased density?** Strength training, for example, can have a significant impact on bone density.

◆ **Will the advertiser supply you with the details of the density test?**
When you study all of the results of the DXA tests, you may discover
some undesired surprises.

Marketers can choose whichever bone density results make their product
look good. On the other hand, critics can find results that make the same
products look bad. Almost any product can be shown to have either positive
or negative results depending on the data selected.

That's one reason why scientists don't just rely on bone density tests to
determine if a product is effective. They compare the fracture rates of
people using the product to those who don't; and in certain instances, they
do bone biopsies. They also test patients' blood and urine to determine
bone changes.

It's best that human osteoporosis studies be conducted over a period of
several years; the longer the study, the more convincing it can be. For
example, it's difficult to draw firm conclusions from my test data now
about the effect of alendronate on my bone density. But after a few years
of data gathering, it will be easier.

One problem with many osteoporosis studies is that they don't include
important variables such as the type and amount of exercise the participants
were getting during the study. That's one reason why I decided to be tested
at frequent intervals. By analyzing my own results, I can better determine
the kinds of exercise that are best for various parts of my skeleton. I'm also
able to take into consideration nutritional changes, stress and my overall
health. In other words, I know the variables that might be affecting the
density of my bones.

The next time someone promotes an osteoporosis product with testimonials of how it's helped increase bone density, consider asking for
detailed written documentation of the test results. Ask, too, for written and
preferably published evidence of independent research studies. If they
claim their product has no side effects, find out how they have determined
this and how many people they have tested. Bear in mind that advertisers
seldom disclose the negative points of their product unless they are obliged
to do so by the government. Objectivity is often compromised whenever
financial gain from a product is involved.

Many factors can affect bone density including, diet, menstrual history,
certain medications, minerals, vitamins, illnesses, amount of exercise, and
type of exercise. You should consider all of them and get a complete
picture of your particular situation when drawing conclusions from bone
density tests.

Conclusions from This Four-year Study

After reviewing the tables of all my results in this chapter, it appears to me that **site-specific, weight-bearing or weight-resisting exercise may be my best defense against bone loss**, as long as I maintain a healthy diet. Yoga includes some of these types of exercise; my spine and hip density did improve while I was doing it 2–4 times per week during Period 2. During Period 3, when I stopped doing yoga, the gains either decreased or I lost bone. The most obvious evidence of improvement in my spine occurred during Period 4 when I strength trained using resistance machines, dumbbells and my own body weight.

According to the US Surgeon General's 2004 report, *Bone Health & Osteoporosis* (p 171), "The evidence suggests that the most beneficial activity regimens for bone health include strength-training or resistance-training activities. These activities place levels of loading on bone that are beyond those seen in everyday activities."

When I started weight training, I discovered that the muscles in my hip area were weak, even though I run a mile on most days and do a lot of walking. My trainer told me that unless I lift my legs really high in marching form, running will not work the hip area muscles much. This helped me understand why the density in my femoral neck and trochanter went down considerably during Period 1, unlike the shaft of my leg. Even though my legs got lots of exercise during Period 1, my hips didn't get as much.

Other deductions I've made from my test results include:

◆ **The best way for me to fight osteoporosis is to combine a variety of preventive measures**—drug therapy, strength training, weight-bearing activities, good nutrition, soy products, vitamin and mineral supplements when necessary, etc. The combination of all of these steps probably led to my increase in bone density at a time just after menopause (period 4) when my bone density would normally be dropping significantly.

Another reason for taking several preventive steps is to assure that bones remain strong and resistant to fracture. Researchers are not yet able to measure bone strength in humans, nor are they certain as to how to increase it, but animal studies suggest that exercise and mechanical stimulation increase bone strength and density. Combining several preventive measures seems to be the best way of avoiding fractures; in my case, at least, it's helped me avoid them.

◆ **I've received several health benefits from taking preventive steps against osteoporosis**—increased muscle strength, more energy, better posture, more resistance to muscle injuries, increased balance, and no doubt better general health.

Analyzing my bone density results has given me an optimistic view of my future. When I see clinical evidence that my density can improve at a time when it would normally decline, I realize that I have considerable control over the health of my bones. Although every person is different, you too, can take steps to help control your own bone health destiny.

18

How to Help Prevent Osteoporosis and Broken Bones

Five factors that affect your skeleton and that you can control are:

◆ **Diet**

◆ **Physical activity and site-specific exercise**

◆ **Medications**

◆ **Posture**

◆ **Bone-depleting habits**: smoking and high alcohol consumption

Other variables such as age, gender, body size, ethnicity, and heredity also affect your bones, but they are beyond your control. Nevertheless, if you pay attention to the factors that you can change, you can help prevent osteoporosis. For further information on risk factors that you can't control, see Chapter 3.

Even if you already have osteoporosis, it's never too late to improve bone quality or strengthen the muscles protecting your bones; nor is it ever too late to take steps to prevent falls.

The following sections review what you can do to prevent osteoporosis and broken bones. Some new information is included.

Diet

Your bones need more than calcium to grow and be strong. They also need protein, vitamins D, A, C, B_6, B_9, B_{12}, K, magnesium, phosphorous, zinc, boron, manganese, copper, potassium, silica, fluoride and essential fatty acids. Plant-derived estrogens called isoflavones are also helpful for maintaining bone mass, but they are not essential. Isoflavones are mostly found in soybean products (see Chapter 9).

The safest and most natural way to get bone nutrients is by eating a varied diet of nutritious food including fruits, vegetables, seafood, poultry, meat, eggs, dairy products, nuts, beans and whole grains. If dietary restrictions prevent you from getting enough of the required nutrients, supplements can be useful. However, in excess quantities, supplementary vitamins and minerals can do more harm than good, especially when they're taken alone.

For example, excess quantities of vitamin A can cause reduced bone density as well as birth defects and liver abnormalities.

In her book *Better Bones, Better Body* (p. 248), nutritionist Susan Brown, PhD says, "Using high doses of calcium in the face of magnesium deficiency can contribute to a depositing of calcium in the joints promoting arthritis, in the kidney contributing to kidney stones, or in the arteries contributing to vascular and heart disease." Excessive amounts of calcium can also lead to Alzheimer's disease and learning disorders (*Calcium Hypothesis of Aging and Dementia, Volume 747*, Annals of the New York Academy of Sciences).

Fad diets that focus only on one food group can also lead to bone loss by not providing all of the necessary bone nutrients. High protein diets can draw calcium out of the bones, resulting in bone loss. This is because calcium is required for protein metabolism. Nonetheless, protein is required for building bones. In addition, meat, fish and mollusks are the best sources of zinc and vitamin B_{12}, two important nutrients for bone formation.

Excessive dieting or "yo-yo" dieting can also cause bone loss. In her book *Strong Women Strong Bones* (p 54), Miriam Nelson, PhD, states that frequent cycles of losing and regaining fifteen or more pounds increases your risk of osteoporosis. Rapid weight loss is especially detrimental. You can counter these effects by losing weight gradually and by doing aerobic exercise and strength training.

In summary, **eat a well-balanced diet, avoid excessive supplementation, and try to get your bone nutrients mainly from food**. Chapters 8 and 9 explain how to get the right amount of bone nutrients and include charts indicating the best food sources of various vitamins and minerals.

Physical Activity

Sedentary lifestyles can lead to bone loss. Physicians have observed that patients who are paralyzed or who are bedridden have less bone on x-rays. Comparisons of bone density in patients before and after a month of bed rest have also indicated that people who are inactive are more likely to lose bone than those who have active lifestyles. (*Osteoporosis Handbook*, p. 72, by Sydney Bonnick, MD)

Physical activity, on the other hand, helps build and maintain bone. For example, one study in Finland compared the bone density of the playing arm of adult women tennis players with their non-dominant arm. The bone density of the playing arm averaged 12–16 percent higher in the playing arm. (Kannus et al, Ann Intern Med, 1995, Jul 1;123[1]; 27-31)

Walking is a safe, excellent general form of exercise, which offers cardiovascular benefits; it's an ideal way to start exercising if you've been sick or are out of shape. However, walking is not sufficient for building bone and preventing bone loss throughout your body. Other exercise that targets the spine, hips, and wrists is also required for building bone in these areas, which are susceptible to fractures.

In her *Osteoporosis Handbook* (p 74), Sydney Lou Bonnick, MD, FACP, states "Exercise is site specific. If you want a strong spine, you must exercise the spine. If you want strong legs, you must exercise the legs."

What type of exercise is best? On page 171 of *Bone Health and Osteoporosis*, the US Surgeon General states, "Physical activity to specifically benefit bone health should involve loading (stressing) the skeleton. As a result, weight-bearing activities such as walking should be included in an optimal physical activity regimen. . . . Moreover, the evidence suggests that **the most beneficial physical activity regimens for bone health include strength-training or resistance training activities**."

In his book *Stand Tall* (p 115), Morris Notelovitz, MD, PhD, a pioneer in the clinical use of densitometers, states, "Study after study has shown that weight training may be the best exercise for increasing bone density. The increase is directly proportional to the amount of stress applied." One preliminary study at his clinic found that after fifteen months, postmenopausal women participating in muscle strengthening exercises on Nautilus equipment achieved the same improvement in bone density as women taking hormone therapy.

Weight training can enhance the effects of drug therapy. After I started to strength train while taking Fosamax (alendronate), my bone density showed a greater increase. To get maximum benefit from osteoporosis medication, I had to do more than walk and run.

Besides maintaining bone, exercise can improve balance, an ability that often starts to decline in people in their mid-forties. The better your sense of balance, the less likely you are to fall; the less you fall, the less likely you are to break a bone. One-legged yoga poses and tandem walking can help people improve their balance. ("In tandem" means "in single file; one behind the other.") Walking with your feet directly in front of each other as if they were on a balance beam is tandem walking. When you do this, make sure that you have something to grab onto in case you lose your balance. You can test your balance simply by standing with one foot in front of each other while standing next to a counter so you can catch yourself if necessary. If this is easy, try doing it with your eyes closed.

Even if you don't do exercises specifically geared to improving balance, you can help maintain it by doing general exercise and keeping active. Just as our bones need a variety of nutrients to remain strong, our bones and muscles need a variety of exercise. If you want to help prevent bone loss, spend at least two or three hours per week doing exercises that involve your entire body—shoulders, arms, wrists, back, abdomen, buttocks, hips, legs, ankles and feet. In addition to the exercises, include physical activities such as grocery shopping, housework, gardening, hiking, sports, dancing, etc. In other words, don't spend your life just sitting in a chair and lying in bed.

One of the advantages of bone density tests is that they can often indicate which areas of the skeleton are getting the least and most exercise. For example, you can determine whether a baseball pitcher is right- or left-handed by comparing the results of bone density tests of both arms. The arm with the highest density will be the one the person uses the most.

Likewise, your bone density tests may point out areas of weakness in your spine and hip that need more exercise than others. **In order to determine your areas of weakness and fully benefit from your bone density tests, you must get a written copy of the test report.** It should include the densities of the various areas that were tested. A general summary of your bone density is not sufficient.

Before you start an exercise program, consult your physician, especially if you have heart problems, osteoporosis, or are recovering from surgery or an illness. Don't do anything mentioned in this book, without first consulting an appropriate professional. If you have osteoporosis, ask your doctor to refer you to a physical therapist who can recommend safe types of exercise for you.

If exercise is not done properly, it can do more harm than good. Two important precautions are to start gradually and avoid exercising injured muscles unless you are under the supervision of a physical therapist or other health professional. If you decide to do strength training, have a trainer check your form and show you how to use the weights and resistance machines. Whether you're practicing yoga, weight lifting or exercising in general, always have a qualified professional teach you how to use the equipment and have proper form.

Any type of exercise can cause serious injury if not done correctly; when done right it can improve your overall health as well as strengthen your bones and muscles.

Why are strong muscles important? They can help protect your bones from fracturing if you fall or get into an accident. The Surgeon General's report *Bone Health and Osteoporosis* (p 130) states, "Muscle strengthening reduces the risk of fractures by improving balance, mobility, and speed of movement, each of which helps to prevent or reduce the severity of falls."

In brief, if you want to help prevent osteoporosis, you must maintain an active lifestyle and do different exercises that target all areas of your body. In addition, get a bone density test of your hip and spine if you are at risk of osteoporosis.

Medications

Some drugs can cause bone loss because they decrease calcium absorption, inhibit bone formation, or increase urinary calcium excretion. These medications include anticonvulsants, diuretics, antacids with aluminum, thyroid medication and steroids like cortisone and prednisone. If you take them, ask your doctor if your bone density should be monitored while you're on treatment. If there are side effects to your bones, find out what you can do to counter the loss. **Never change the dose or stop taking the medication without first consulting your doctor**. See Chapter 3 for a more detailed list of pharmaceuticals that can lead to bone loss.

On the other hand, some drugs can help build bone or prevent bone loss. These include Actonel® (risedronate), Evista® (raloxiphene), Fosamax® (alendronate), Boniva® (ibandronate), Miacalcin Nasal Spray® (calcitonin), Forteo® (teriparatide), Didronel PMO® (cyclical etidronate), Protelos® (strontium ranelate) and hormone replacement therapy drugs. Your doctor and the websites listed in the appendix can provide information on these osteoporosis medications. Availability depends on your country of residence.

If you decide to use a bone-building drug, don't use it as an excuse for inactivity. It's just as important to exercise and eat healthy food when you are taking an osteoporosis medication as when you are not.

Posture

The way you stand and sit affects your bones and your balance. People who get into the habit of slumping, can gradually develop a hunched back, even if they don't have osteoporosis. Slumping is associated with weak back muscles. If you want to avoid looking like you have osteoporosis, work on strengthening your back muscles and improving your posture. Chapter 7, "Posture and Osteoporosis," provides tips on having a youthful posture.

Bone-Depleting Habits

Smoking lowers estrogen levels, interferes with calcium absorption and inhibits the growth of bone-building cells. As a result, smokers have an increased risk of developing osteoporosis. The more they smoke, the greater their risk of low bone mass. According to the US Surgeon General, the nicotine and cadmium found in cigarettes can have a direct toxic effect on bone cells. Several studies have linked smoking to higher fracture risk. (*Bone Health and Osteoporosis,* pp 139 & 140, 2004)

Another bone-depleting habit is excessive alcohol consumption. It impairs calcium absorption through the intestines and it affects the liver's ability to activate vitamin D. Another problem with drinking is that it can affect your balance and make you more likely to fall.

In his book *Stand Tall* (p 49), Dr. Morris Notelovitz suggests limiting yourself to no more than one or two drinks per day (One standard drink = 12 oz beer, 5 oz wine, or 1.5 oz of 80 proof liquor). He also advises that you avoid any alcohol within an hour or two of eating calcium-rich foods or taking a calcium supplement, and that you avoid alcohol altogether if you have low bone mass. According to Notelovitz "even moderate drinking has been found to interfere with the bone remodeling cycle, reduce thickness of trabecular bone and interfere with proper bone mineralization." (See Chapter 4 for an explanation of bone terminology.)

In summary, if you'd like to help prevent osteoporosis and avoid bone fractures,

◆ Limit your intake of alcohol and avoid smoking.
◆ Stand and sit tall with good posture.
◆ Find out if your medications might be affecting your bones, and use osteoporosis drugs if appropriate.
◆ Keep active and do a variety of exercises that target your entire body. Use your bone density tests to motivate you to exercise and to determine which areas of your skeleton have the lowest bone mass and need the most physical activity. Do additional site-specific exercises for the weak areas.
◆ Eat well-balanced meals, and take supplements if you can't get an adequate amount of bone nutrients from food.

Ten Major Causes of Falls and Broken Bones

No matter what your age or how strong your bones are, you should take precautions to avoid falls. Awareness of hazards can help prevent broken bones. Below are ten major causes of falls:

1. **Uneven sidewalks, unexpected steps or stairs**. Uneven sidewalks should be repaired with asphalt or another material. Buildings, homes and outdoor areas should be designed so that stairs or steps are easily visible. If this isn't possible, brightly colored adhesive tape applied to the outer edge of stairs can make them easier to see.

2. **Liquid spills on the floor**. These should be wiped up immediately.

3. **Stairways with no railings**. Every stairway should have at least one railing. When carrying items up stairs, try to have one hand free so it can grasp the railing. It's better to make several trips up stairs than to risk losing your balance with your arms full of bags and boxes. Grab-bars in showers and on bathroom walls are also good safety features.

4. **Clutter on the floor**. Move clutter, toys and furniture away from where you walk.

5. **Unstable or weak ladders.** Discard old rickety ladders and replace them with sturdy ones. Position ladders so they are close to the objects that you are trying to reach. Many accidents happen when people lean and turn to reach for distant objects instead of simply repositioning the ladder. Use spotters when possible.

6. **Ice on the sidewalk and ground.** Unfortunately it's not always possible to cover ice with gritty substances like salt. Therefore, wear shoes with good traction when outdoors in freezing weather.

7. **Throw rugs**. These are especially dangerous on slippery floors and should be removed, especially when older people are in the room. Carpeting should be tacked down and secure.

8. **Electrical and telephone cords and cables**. Tuck them out of the way or fasten them to the wall so you don't trip over them.

9. **Poor lighting**. Install lighting in stairwells, corridors and garages. Use night-lights in bathrooms and halls, and have flashlights available.

10 **Shoes with slippery soles, high heels or no heel support (clogs)**. Wear low-heeled shoes with good support and flexible, nonskid soles whenever possible. Proper footwear is important for preventing falls.

More Tips for Avoiding Falls and Fractures

1. **Place your heel down first when you walk, not your toe**. This can help you avoid tripping. The muscles and tendons around our ankles can become weak with age, making it more difficult for us to raise the front of our foot as we walk. To keep your feet and ankle muscles in shape,

practice walking with the heel down first and the toes facing upward followed by the balls of your feet gradually touching the ground. Also, include toe raises and ankle-strengthening exercises in your exercise routine.

2. **Use a walker or cane if you're unsteady on your feet.** This makes some people feel self-conscious, but it's better than falling.

3. **Store often-used items in easy-to-reach places** so that you don't have to climb on a chair or stepladder to reach them.

4. **Wear hip protectors if you're at high risk of falls.** Hip protectors use either foam pads or rigid shells made of durable plastic designed to protect the bone from a direct impact. The hip protector works by diverting energy from a sideways fall away from the protruding bone (trochanter) onto the surrounding soft tissue. Three basic types of hip protectors are:

   a. underwear with sewn-in shields or pads—the most popular type.

   b. underwear with pockets that hold shock guards in place.

   c. a hip protector belt worn outside of the garment.

   All three types can be worn over disposable pants, if necessary.

   Sweden and Australia are two countries in which hip protectors are widely used for fracture prevention in the elderly. In fact in Sweden, the government provides people at risk for fractures with hip protectors because they've found this to be a cost-effective way of preventing fractures.

   For maximum benefit, hip protectors should be worn all the time, not just in risky situations such as icy weather. Most falls happen right inside the home. In addition, the pads or shields must be properly positioned. Hip protectors can be purchased at medical supply stores or on the Internet.

How to Help Others Maintain Strong Bones & Good Health

This chapter has provided tips on how individuals can avoid osteoporosis. It's important to take care of our own health, but we should go beyond ourselves. There are things we as a society can do to help others have strong bones and good health. Here are some suggestions:

◆ Make physical education in schools a priority and encourage children to participate in sports. Some schools have significantly reduced their physical education and sports programs in order to cut down on expenses. Exercise is a key factor in building peak bone mass and in preventing heart disease, diabetes and obesity. Exercise also helps improve concentration and mental health. For those reasons, we should help children form good, lifelong fitness habits by supporting physical education programs.

◆ Replace junk food in school vending machines with nutritious food.

◆ Include nutrition as part of the school curriculum.

◆ Discourage children and adults from smoking. Point out to them that the people they're trying to impress by looking cool probably won't be by their bedside if they end up in the hospital with an illness brought on by smoking.

◆ Encourage seniors to be active. Instead of doing everything for them, let them participate in daily activities such as cooking, gardening, house cleaning, grocery shopping, etc. Include daily exercise sessions and physical therapy at adult day health care facilities. Have well-organized transportation programs that allow seniors to get out of their homes.

◆ Instead of focusing on how to pay for drugs, let's concentrate more on how to eliminate the need for them.

◆ Encourage people to take responsibility for their health. Patients must develop good health habits, but medical professionals can help by encouraging patients to study their own medical reports and take preventive steps to improve their conditions.

Many countries are experiencing a health care crisis, brought on in large part by poor nutrition, inadequate exercise, smoking, excess alcohol consumption, and over medication. This is why some of the highest rates of osteoporosis are found in the most technologically advanced countries. Instead of spending millions of dollars in treating patients' ailments; we should invest in people who are committed to preventive health care. For example, we need bone density test centers that educate their patients on how to prevent osteoporosis. Currently such centers are hard to find in many countries.

Osteoporosis is not an inevitable part of aging. If you maintain a positive attitude and follow the preventive guidelines in this book, you can improve the strength of your bones; in doing so, you will also improve your general health.

Websites

Osteoporosis Websites

www.nof.org National Osteoporosis Foundation

www.osteofound.org International Osteoporosis Foundation (IOF)

www.nos.org.uk National Osteoporosis Society

www.osteo.org National Institutes of Health, Osteoporosis and Related Bone Diseases–National Resource Center

www.cdc.gov/powerfulbones Powerful Bones Powerful Girls, National Bone Health Campaign

www.bonezone.org.uk Fun for kids and teenagers

www.surgeongeneral.gov/library/bonehealth

www.susanbrownphd.com

www.avoidboneloss.com

www.nlm.nih.gov/medlineplus/osteoporosis.html By the US National Library of Medicine and the National Institutes of Health

www.courses.washington.edu/bonephys Osteoporosis & Bone Physiology

www.iscd.org International Society for Clinical Densitometry

www.osteoporosis.org.au Osteoporosis Australia

www.osteoporosis.ca Osteoporosis Society of Canada

www.osteofound.org/latinoamerica IOF Latin America

www.osteofound.org/mena IOF Middle East & North Africa

www.apof.org Asian Pacific Osteoporosis Foundation (Hong Kong)

www.anzbms.org.au Australia and New Zealand Bone & Mineral Society

www.anzbms.org.au Belgium Association for Osteoporosis Patients

www.china-osteofound.org China Osteoporosis Foundation

www.grio.org Group of Research and Osteoporosis Information (France)

www.bfo-aktuell.de Bundesselbsthilfeverband für Osteoporose e. V.

www.isbmr.org Indian Society of Bone & Mineral Research

www.irishosteoporosis.ie Irish Osteoporosis Society

www.aslo.lu Osteoporosis Association of Luxembourg

www.osteoporosestichting.nl Osteoporosis Foundation of Netherlands

www.bones.org.nz Osteoporosis New Zealand

www.osteoporosissoc.org.sg Osteoporosis Society (Singapore)

www.osteoporosis.org.za National Osteoporosis Foundation of South Africa

www.fhoemo.com Hispanic Foundation of Osteoporosis and Metabolic Diseases

www.aecos.es Spanish Association Against Osteoporosis

www.knochenundmineralstoffwechsel.at Austrian Society for Bone & Mineral Research

Osteoporosis Drug Websites

www.actonel.com

www.evista.com

www.forteo.com

www.fosamax.com

www.calcitonin.com

www.myboniva.com

www.servier.com/pro/identification.asp (site for Protelos based in France)

www.servier.co.uk/patients/osteoporosis.asp (based in UK)

Bibliography

Books and Booklets

Golding, Lawrence & Scott. *AFPA Fitness Professional's Guide to Musculoskeletal Anatomy and Human Movement.* Monterey, CA: Healthy Learning, 2003.

Allanore, Yannick, *Ostéoporose et Autres Ostéopathies.* Paris: Editions Estem, 1998.

Bassey, Joan & Dinan, Susie. *Exercise for Strong Bones,* London: Carroll & Brown Publishers, 2001.

Bonnick, Sydney Lou *The Osteoporosis Handbook.* Lanham, MD: Taylor Trade Publishing, 1994.

Bonnick, Sydney Lou. *Bone Densitometry for Technologists.* Totowa, NJ: Humana Press, 2002.

Bissenger, Margie. *Osteoporosis: An Exercise Guide.* Workfit Consultants, 1998.

Brown, Susan E. *Better Bones, Better Body.* Los Angeles: Keats Publishing, 2000.

Colbin, Annemarie. *Food & Our Bones.* New York: Plume, 1998.

Comston, Juliet. *Ostéoporose: Guide de Médecine Famliale.* London: Dorling Kindersley, Marabout, 1999.

Cooperman, Tod et al. *Guide to Buying Vitamins & Supplements.* White Plains, NY: ConsumerLab.com, 2003.

Cosman, Felicia. *What Your Doctor May Not Tell You About Osteoporosis.* New York: Warner Books, 2003.

Daniels, Diane. *Exercises for Osteoporosis.* New York: Hatherleigh Press, 2000.

Disterhoft, John et al. *Calcium Hypothesis of Aging and Dementia.* New York: New York Academy of Sciences, 1994.

Finocchi, Joanne et al. *PDR Monthly Prescribing Guide.* Montvale, NJ: Thomson PDR, 2005.

Fuchs, Nan Kathryn. *Basic Health Publications User's Guide to Calcium & Magnesium.* North Bergen, NJ: Basic Health Publications, 2002.

Gaby, Alan. *Preventing & Reversing Osteoporosis.* New York: Prima Publishing, 1994.

Gates, Rhonda & Whipple, Beverly. *Outwitting Osteoporosis.* Hillsboro, OR: Beyond Woods Publishing, 2003.

Genest, Lyse & Le Rouzès, Monique. *Sauvez Vos Os.* Outrement, Québec: Les Editions Quebecor, 1994.

Gray, Henry. *Gray's Anatomy: The Anatomical Basis of Medicine and Surgery, Thirty-Eighth Edition.* Churchill Livingstone, 1995.

Harvard Medical School. *Boosting Bone Strength.* 2003.

Hodgson, Stephen. *Mayo Clinic on Osteoporosis.* Rochester, NY: Mayo Clinic, 2003.

Lee, Deborah. *Osteoporosis: A Woman's Guide to Natural and Safe Prevention Therapies.* Pleasant Grove, UT, 1997.

Levin, Pamela. *Perfect Bones.* Berkeley, CA: Celestial Arts, 2002.

Ley, Beth M. *How to Fight Osteoporosis and Win.* Aliso Viejo, CA, 1996.

Lineback, Karena Thek. *Osteo Pilates.* Franklin Lakes, NJ: New Page Books, 2003.

MacWilliam, Lyle. *Comparative Guide to Nutritional Supplements: 3rd Edition.* Vernon, BC, Northern Dimensions. 2003.

Maddern, Jan. *Yoga Builds Bones:* Gloucester, MA: Fair Winds Press, 2000.

Marmot, Michael. *The Status Syndrome.* New York: Times Books. 2004.

McIlwain, Harris & Fulghum Bruce, Debra. *Reversing Osteopenia.* New York: Henry Holt & Co. 2004.

McIlwain, Harris & Fulghum Bruce, Debra. *The Osteoporosis Cure.* New York: Avon Books: 1998.

Meeks, Sara. *Walk Tall: An Exercise Program for the Prevention & Treatment of Osteoporosis.* Gainesville, FL: Triad Publishing Co. , 1999.

Netter, Frank, H. *Atlas of Human Anatomy.* Summit, NJ, Ciba-Geigy Corp., 1989.

National Osteoporosis Foundation. *Boning up on Osteoporosis.* 2003.

Nelson, Miriam E. *Strong Women, Strong Bones:* New York, Berkeley Publishing, 2000.

Notelovitz, Morris, *Stand Tall: Every Woman's Guide to Preventing and Treating Osteoporosis.* Gainesville, FL: Triad Publishing Co., 1998.

O'Connor, Carolyn & Perkins, Sharon. *Osteoporosis for Dummies.* Hoboken, NJ: Wiley Publishing, 2005.

Plant, Jane & Tidey, Gill. *Understanding, Preventing & Overcoming Osteoporosis.* London: Virgin Books, 2003.

Prevention Magazine, *Doctor's Book of Home Remedies for Stronger Bones.* Emmaus, PA: Rodale Inc. 2000.

Richards, Ann & Levine, Richard. *I'm Not Slowing Down: Winning my Battle with Osteoporosis.* New York: Dutton, 2003.

Root, Leon. *Beautiful Bones Without Hormones.* New York: Gotham Books. 2004.

Savard, Marie, *How to Save Your Own Life.* New York: Warner Books, 2000.

Solomon, Neil. *Soy Smart Health.* Orem, Utah: Woodland Publishing, 2004.

Sparrowe, Linda & Patricia Walden. *Yoga for Healthy Bones.* Boston: Shambhala Publications, 2004.

US Public Health Service. *Bone Health and Osteoporosis: A Report by the Surgeon General.* Honolulu: University Press of the Pacific, 2005.

Winters-Stone, Kerri. *Action Plan for Osteoporosis.* Champaign, IL: Human Kinetics, 2005.

Wolf, Sidney et al. *Worst Pills Best Pills.* New York: Pocket Books, 2005.

Journals and Magazines

American Family Physician. Leawood, KS: American Academy of Family Physicians.

American Journal of Clinical Nutrition. Bethesda, MD: American Society for Clinical Nutrition.

American Journal of Family Practice. Montvale, NJ: Dowden Health Media.

American Journal of Medicine. Washington DC: Elsevier.

American Journal of Nursing (AJN). New York, Lippincott Williams & Wilkins.

American Journal of Sports Medicine (AJSM). Rosemont, IL: American Orthopaedic Society for Sports Medicine.

Annals of Biomedical Engineering. Landover, MD: Biomedical Engineering Society.

Annals of Internal Medicine. Philadelphia: American College of Physicians.

Annals of the New York Academy of Sciences. New York: New York Academy of Sciences.

Arthritis & Rheumatism. Danvers, MA: American College of Rheumatology.

British Medical Journal (BMJ). London: British Medical Association.

Fitness Mind, Body & Spirit. New York: Meredith Corporation.

Health. Birmingham, AL: Health Magazine.

Journal of Clinical Densitometry. Totowa, NJ: Humana Press.

Journal of the American College of Nutrition. Clearwater, FL: American College of Nutrition.

Journal of the American Dietetic Association. Philadelphia. Elsevier.

Journal of the American Medical Association (JAMA). Chicago: American Medical Association.

Journal of Bone and Mineral Research. Washington DC: American Society for Bone & Mineral Research.

The Journal of Bone and Joint Surgery. Rosemont, IL: The Journal of Bone and Joint Surgery, Inc.

Medicine and Science in Sports and Exercise: Ambler, PA: Lippincott Williams and Wilkins.

Lancet. London: Elsevier Ltd.

New England Journal of Medicine. Boston: Massachusetts Medical Society.

Nurse Week. San Jose, CA: Nurse Week Publishing.

Nursing Weekly Magazine: Reading, MA: Gente Media.

Nursing 2005. Ambler, PA: Lippincott Williams & Wilkins.

Osteoporosis International. Heidelberg: Springer-Verlag London Ltd.

Physical Therapy. Alexandria, VA. American Physical Therapy Association.

Prevention. Emmaus, PA: Rodale Inc.

RN. Montvale, NJ: RN Magazine.

Yoga Journal. San Francisco: Yoga Journal.

Index

Actonel 92, 95, 96
age 13, 110, 111, 161
AI 69, 74, 75
alcohol 16, 61, 162
alendronate (Fosamax) 87-90, 92-96, 39, 143, 144, 147, 152-154
alignment problems 118, 119
amenorrhea 17, 84
anorexia nervosa 16, 84
antacids 18, 62, 72
AP spine 23
arthritis 16, 17, 42, 63, 71, 72
astronauts 28, 97, 98

back strengthening exercises 29, 35
balance exercises 29, 40
bisphosphonates 92, 95
blood clots 91, 95
blood tests 116, 133
BMD 101-104, 140-142, 145-147
bone
    collagen 10, 116
    cortical 24-26
    density 9-12, 101-127, 139-145
    remodeling 25, 26, 116
    strength 9-12, 98
    terminology 21-26
    turnover 25, 87, 116
bone density reports 101-104, 124, 125, 129-132
bone density tests 101, 105-115, 117-132, 139-151
bone-loading activities 34-36
bone marker tests 116
bone marrow 23, 77
bone mineral density (BMD) 101, 104

bone turnover tests 116
bone-depleting habits 162
Boniva 92, 95
boron 68, 75
bulimia 15, 84

caffeine 16, 61, 62
calcitonin 95
calcium 53-68
    absorption 59-61
    component in bone 10, 12
    coral 64, 65
    determining content 55-58
    food sources 55-58
    guidelines for consumption 62-63
    recommended intake 6, 54
    harmful effects of excess 63, 64
    magnesium balance 63, 71, 72, 158
    supplements 58-60, 64, 65
calcium carbonate 53, 58-60, 62, 65
calcium citrate 59, 60, 62, 142
calcium gluconate 60
calcium lactate 59
calcium phosphate 59
certified trainers 37
collagen 10, 12, 116
compact bone 25
compression fractures 31, 47, 49, 118
coral calcium 64, 65
cortical bone 24-26
corticosteroids 17, 116, 121, 127, 161

dairy products 55, 59, 65, 66, 76, 86
densitometer 106, 107, 109, 122, 125, 150, 152
DEXA 105

Didrocal 95
dieting 15, 83, 158
doctor's order 128
dowager's hump 49
DRI 69
drugs
  Actonel (risedronate) 88, 92, 93, 95, 96
  bisphosphonates 92, 95
  bone-depleting 17, 18
  Boniva (ibandronate) 88, 92, 93, 95, 161
  Didrocal (etidronate) 95
  estrogen 4, 13-17, 67, 75, 79, 84, 89, 90, 94, 95
  Evista (raloxifene) 95, 96
  Forteo (teriparatide) 95, 96
  Fosamax (alendronate) 87-90, 93, 92-96, 140, 143, 144, 152
  hormones 90-92, 94, 95
  ipriflavone 79
  Miacalcin (calcitonin) 95, 161
  Prempro 91, 95
  progesterone 91, 92
  Protelos (strontium ranelate) 95, 96

dual energy x-ray absorptiometry 4, 7, 105, 118
DV 69, 74, 77
DXA 4, 7, 105-107, 112-119, 150
DXA images 7, 8, 109, 118, 119
DXA tests 105-118, 126-128, 139

EAR 69, 75
estrogen 4, 13-17, 67, 75, 79, 84, 89, 90, 94, 95
etidronate 95, 161
Evista 95, 96
exercise 27- 46, 142- 144, 158-161
  resistance 28, 31, 32, 35-38, 143
  walking 28, 29, 159
  weight-bearing 28, 34, 142, 155
  weight-training 31, 32, 37, 38, 143, 144, 155

yoga 30, 31, 33, 35-37, 39, 50, 143, 144, 155

female athlete triad 17
femoral neck 21, 23, 108, 119, 125, 145, 147, 149-152
femur 21, 26, 130
fiber 61, 85
FIT 88, 90
fitness machines 33
fluoride 68, 82
folic acid 68, 77, 78
Forteo 95, 96
Fosamax 87-90, 93, 92-96, 140, 143, 144, 152, 161
fracture prevention 163-165
fracture risk 8, 10, 21, 95, 102, 119

greater trochanter 21, 108

height loss 15
heredity 14
hip
  axis 119, 125
  fracture 16, 54, 77, 82
  terminology 21-23
hip protectors 164, 165
HMO 126, 137
hormone replacement therapy 91, 95
hormones 90-92, 94, 95

ibandronate 88, 92, 93, 95, 161
ipriflavone 79
IU 68-71, 81

Juvent 97-99

kyphoplasty 49
kyphosis 49

lactose intolerance 66
lumbar spine 8, 22, 23, 108, 109, 114, 115, 117, 118, 125, 141, 145, 146, 148, 150, 153

lumbar vertebrae 23, 108, 109, 125,
       141, 145
magnesium 62-65, 68, 71-73
medical reports 133-136, 165
medication (see drugs) 17, 18, 87-96,
       161, 162
menopause 13-15, 89, 90, 102, 103,
       110, 112, 143-145, 161
Miacalcin 95, 161
milk 54-56, 65-67, 70, 71, 76-78, 86

nutrition 54, 55, 67-81, 83-85

osteoarthritis 2, 47, 83, 94
osteoblasts 25, 67, 74, 77
osteoclasts 25, 26, 74, 95
osteopenia 7, 89, 101-104, 109, 110,
       145-151
osteoporosis
    basic information 4-6
    definition 2, 4
    diagnosis 8, 101-103, 106-112
    in men 110
    medications 87-96, 161
    secondary 17
    specialist 120, 127, 140, 152, 153
oxalates 60, 61

PA spine 23
pDXA 105
Percent Daily Value 6, 55
peripheral QCT 106
physical activity 34-43, 158-160
phytates 60, 61
phytoestrogens 79
posture 49-52
pQCT 106
Prempro 91, 95
progesterone 91, 92
protein 10, 61, 81, 157, 158
Protelos 95, 96

QCT 106, 107
quantitative computed tomography
       106

quantitative ultrasound 105, 106
QUS 105

radiographic absorptiometry 106
raloxifene 95
RDA 69
resistance exercises 28, 31, 32, 35-38,
       45, 143
resorption 25, 67, 95
risedronate 88, 92, 93, 95
risk factors 13-19, 103, 110, 157
running 29, 30

savvy patient 130-132
shaft 21, 22, 119, 142, 155
smoking 15, 162, 166
sodium 17, 61, 62
soy products 79, 80, 90, 143, 155
steroids 17, 19, 110, 111
strength training 31-38, 143, 144, 155,
       158, 160
strontium ranelate 95, 161
supplements 53-82, 157
swimming 28, 29, 40
SXA 105

technologists 114, 120-124
teriparatide 95, 161
testimonials 153, 154
testosterone 4, 13
thoracic kyphosis 49
thyroid 17, 91, 95
tolerable upper intake levels 68, 69
trabecular bone 23-26, 98, 162
trainer 31-33, 36-38, 129
    certified 37
trochanter 21, 22, 25, 108, 142, 147,
       149-152
trochanteric region 21, 23, 108
T-score 8, 101-104, 108, 109, 127,
       145-151

UL 69, 72, 76
upper limits of vitamins and minerals
       68

ultrasound 105, 106, 122, 123
urine tests 116
USP 62

vertebrae 23-26, 107-109, 119, 125,
        141, 145, 150
vertebroplasty 49
vibrating platform therapy 5, 97-99
vibration therapy 97-99
vitamins 67-74, 77, 78, 81
  A 68, 69, 81, 158
  C 68
  B_{12} 67, 68, 77, 78
  E 68
  D 65-71
  K 67, 68, 73, 74
  recommended intakes 68
volunteering 40, 43, 47, 48

walking 28, 29, 159
ward's area 23, 149
weight 83-86
weight training 31-33, 37, 38, 143,
        155, 159
weight-bearing activities 5, 34, 45,
        155, 159
weight-bearing exercise 28, 34, 142,
        155, 159
wild yam cream 91, 92

yoga 30, 31, 33, 35-37, 39, 50, 143,
        144, 155

zinc 67, 68, 76
Z-score 101, 103, 104, 148, 149

Other Books by RENÉE NEWMAN
Graduate Gemologist (GIA)

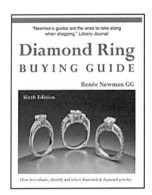

Diamond Ring Buying Guide
How to Evaluate, Identify and Select
Diamonds & Diamond Jewelry

"**An entire course on judging diamonds in 156 pages of well-organized information**. . . .The photos are excellent . . . Clear and concise, it serves as a check-list for the purchase and mounting of a diamond . . . another fine update in a series of books that are useful to both the jewelry industry and consumers."
Gems & Gemology

"**A wealth of information** . . . delves into the intricacies of shape, carat weight, color, clarity, setting style, and cut—happily avoiding all industry jargon and keeping explanations streamlined enough so even the first-time diamond buyer can confidently choose a gem."
Booklist

"Succinctly written in a step-by-step, outlined format with plenty of photographs to illustrate the salient points; it could help keep a lot of people out of trouble. Essentially, it is a **fact-filled text devoid of a lot of technical mumbo-jumbo.** This is a definite thumbs up!"
C. R. Beesley, President, American Gemological Laboratories

156 pages, 193 color & b/w photos, 7" X 9", ISBN 0-929975-32-4, US$17.95

Gem & Jewelry Pocket Guide
Small enough to use while shopping locally or abroad

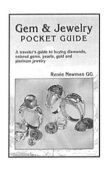

"**Brilliantly planned, painstakingly researched, and beautifully produced** . . . this handy little book comes closer to covering all of the important bases than any similar guides have managed to do. From good descriptions of the most popular gem materials (plus gold and platinum), to jewelry craftsmanship, treatments, gem sources, appraisals, documentation, and even information about U.S. customs for foreign travelers—it is all here. I heartily endorse this wonderful pocket guide."
John S. White, former Curator of Gems & Minerals at the Smithsonian,
Lapidary Journal

"**Short guides don't come better than this**. . . . As always with this author, the presentation is immaculate and each opening displays high-class pictures of gemstones and jewellery." *Journal of Gemmology*

156 pages, 108 color photos, 4½" by 7", ISBN 0-929975-30-8, US$11.95

Available at major bookstores and jewelry supply stores

For more information, see **www.reneenewman.com**

Other Books by RENÉE NEWMAN

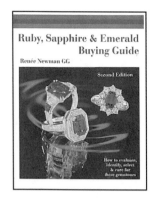

Ruby, Sapphire & Emerald Buying Guide

How to evaluate, identify, and select these gemstones

"**Enjoyable reading . . . profusely illustrated with color photographs** showing not only the beauty of finished jewelry but close-ups and magnification of details such as finish, flaws and fakes . . . Sophisticated enough for professionals to use . . . highly recommended . . . **Newman's guides are the ones to take along when shopping.**" *Library Journal*

"**Solid, informative and comprehensive** . . . dissects each aspect of ruby and sapphire value in detail . . . a wealth of grading information . . . a definite thumbs-up. There is something here for everyone." C. R. Beesley, President, American Gemological Laboratories, *JCK Magazine*

"**The best produced book on gemstones I have yet seen in this price range** (how is it done?). This is the book for anyone who buys, sells or studies gemstones. This style of book (and similar ones by the same author) is the only one I know which introduces actual trade conditions and successfully combines a good deal of gemmology with them . . . **Buy it, read it, keep it.**" Michael O'Donoghue, *Journal of Gemmology*

164 pages, 178 color & 21 b/w photos, 7" by 9", ISBN 0-929975-33-2, US$19.95

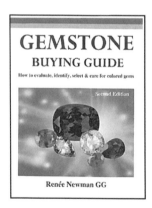

Gemstone Buying Guide

How to Evaluate, Identify and Select Colored Gems

"**Praiseworthy, a beautiful gem-pictorial reference** and a help to everyone in viewing colored stones as a gemologist or gem dealer would. . . . One of the finest collections of gem photographs I've ever seen . . . If you see the book, you will probably purchase it on the spot." *Anglic Gemcutter*

"**A quality Buying Guide** that is recommended for purchase to consumers, gemmologists and students of gemmology—irrespective of their standard of knowledge of gemmology. The information is comprehensive, factual, and well presented. Particularly noteworthy in this book are the quality colour photographs that have been carefully chosen to illustrate the text." *Australian Gemmologist*

"**Beautifully produced.** . . . With colour on almost every opening few could resist this book whether or not they were in the gem and jewellery trade." *Journal of Gemmology*

156 pages, 281 color photos, 7" X 9", ISBN 0-929975-34-0, US$19.95

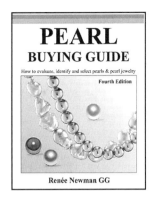

Pearl Buying Guide

How to Evaluate, Identify, Select and Care for Pearls & Pearl Jewelry

"**Copious color photographs** . . . explains how to appraise and distinguish among all varieties of pearls . . . takes potential buyers and collectors through the ins and outs of the pearl world. *Publisher's Weekly*

"**An indispensable guide** to judging [pearl] characteristics, distinguishing genuine from imitation, and making wise choices . . . useful to all types of readers, from the professional jeweler to the average patron . . . **highly recommended.**" *Library Journal*

"A **well written, beautifully illustrated** book designed to help retail customers, jewelry designers, and store buyers make informed buying decisions about the various types of pearls and pearl jewelry. The photos are abundant and well chosen, and the use of a coated stock contributes to the exceptional quality of the reproduction. Consumers also will find this book a source of accurate and easy-to-understand information about a topic that has become increasingly complex."

Gems & Gemology

156 pages, 208 color & b/w photos, 7" by 9", ISBN 0-929975-35-9, US$19.95

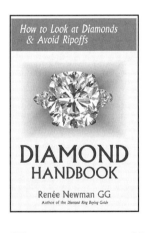

Diamond Handbook

How to Look at Diamonds & Avoid Ripoffs

Provides additional details and photos on clarity & cut, and covers topics not included in the *Diamond Ring Buying Guide* such as:

◆ Antique diamonds and jewelry
◆ Branded diamonds
◆ Diamond certificates, reports, and appraisals
◆ Diamond recutting
◆ Diamond types and synthetic diamonds
◆ Choosing a jeweler, appraiser, and gem lab

"The text covers everything the buyer needs to know, with useful comments on lighting and first-class black and white images that show up features better than those in colour. No other text in current circulation discusses recutting and its possible effects, and the author's discussion of the new topic of branded diamonds conveniently brings together a number of examples of particular cuts peculiar to different firms. . . . Brief and useful notes describe the present position of synthetic gem diamond and treated diamond. Rip-offs are soberly described and sensation avoided. **This is a must for anyone buying, testing or valuing a polished diamond and for students in many fields.**" *Journal of Gemmology*

186 pages, 7 color and 242 b/w photos, 6" x 9", ISBN 0-929975-36-7, US$18.95

Available at major bookstores and jewelry supply stores

Order Form

TITLE	Price Each	Quantity	Total
Osteoporosis Prevention	$15.95		
Gemstone Buying Guide	$19.95		
Ruby, Sapphire & Emerald Buying Guide	$19.95		
Pearl Buying Guide	$19.95		
Diamond Handbook	$18.95		
Diamond Ring Buying Guide	$17.95		
Gem & Jewelry Pocket Guide	$11.95		
		Book Total	
SALES TAX for California residents only **(book total x $.0825)**			
SHIPPING: USA: first book $3.00, each additional copy $1.50 Canada & Mexico - airmail: first book $8.00, ea. addl. $5.00 All other foreign countries - airmail: first book $11.00, ea. addl. $8.00			
TOTAL AMOUNT with tax (if applicable) and shipping (Pay foreign orders with an international money order or a check drawn on a U.S. bank.)		**TOTAL**	

Available at major book stores or by mail

Mail check or money order in U.S. funds

To: International Jewelry Publications
P.O. Box 13384
Los Angeles, CA 90013-0384 USA

Ship to:

Name_____

Address_____

City_____ State or Province_____

Postal or Zip Code_____ Country _____